Hormone Replacement
Therapy Studies

Hormone Replacement Therapy Studies

A Reference Guide

Sara T. Goulden

McFarland & Company, Inc., Publishers
Jefferson, North Carolina, and London

LIBRARY OF CONGRESS CATALOGUING-IN-PUBLICATION DATA

Goulden, Sara T.
    Hormone replacement therapy studies : a reference guide /
Sara T. Goulden.
      p.   cm.
    Includes bibliographical references and index.

    ISBN 0-7864-1683-1 (softcover : 50# alkaline paper)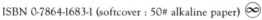

    1. Menopause—Hormone therapy.   I. Title.
RG186.G685 2003
618.1'750651—dc21

                         2003012462

British Library cataloguing data are available

Cover images ©2003 Digital Vision

Manufactured in the United States of America

McFarland & Company, Inc., Publishers
  Box 611, Jefferson, North Carolina 28640
   www.mcfarlandpub.com

Contents

v

Preface

Pharmaceutical companies spend millions of dollars advertising and marketing hormone replacement therapy (HRT). The sales potential is huge and the profit windfalls will be substantial as baby boomers approach menopause. Unfortunately, the information that women are getting from pharmaceutical advertisements about the risks and benefits of HRT is biased and inadequate. The media campaign by the pharmaceutical industry is pervasive. One television commercial shows two middle-aged women discussing all the supposed adverse consequences of not taking HRT. Playing on women's fears of aging and disease, the commercial implies that women who do not take HRT will be at grave risk for blindness, Alzheimer's disease, debilitating heart conditions, sexual problems, and crippling osteoporosis.

Pharmaceutical companies have employed celebrities in their media campaign to sell HRT. Wyeth-Ayerst has enlisted fashion model Lauren Hutton in their television and print promotion of HRT. Hutton, interviewed about "looking and feeling fabulous" in *Parade* magazine (March 2000), attributed her beauty and youthful appearance to estrogen: "It's good for your moods; it's good for your skin. If I had to choose between all my creams and makeup for feeling and looking good, I'd take estrogen." In fact, an information pamphlet about Premarin states that no conclusive evidence supports the idea that estrogen helps to prevent skin from aging. One side effect of estrogen is blotchy skin (hyperpigmentation). A large study, not mentioned in the print advertisement, found no difference in skin collagen between users of estrogen and nonusers (Holland et al., 1994).

Appearing in the same *Parade* magazine was an advertisement with Hutton promoting HRT. The advertisement stated that it was funded by the "Wyeth-Ayerst Women's Health Research Institute," which could lead readers to believe the institute was an impartial foundation for scientific research. Ambiguous and inconclusive phrases ("research has explored," "ongoing research continues to investigate") were used in the ad, but specific results or referenced studies were absent. Like most advertisements promoting HRT, this one stacked the information in favor of the product with no explanation of its downside. When the side effects or risks of HRT are addressed in print ads, the text is small, difficult to read and buried at the bottom of the ad (or even on the back of the page).

A CBS *Sunday Morning* (December 2002) television piece on hormone replacement therapy exemplifies the news media's inadequate and simplistic presentation of health controversies. The reporter presented a brief summary of the results of the Women's Health Initiative (WHI) clinical trial: increased risk of stroke, breast cancer, embolism and heart attack (Writing Group for the Women's Health Initiative Investigators, 2002). However, the reporter marginalized the results of the WHI trial by focusing on the opinions of two women (a doctor and a postmenopausal woman) who favored HRT despite the findings presented by the trial. Minimizing the data from the WHI trial, the reporter injected her own commentary and declared that women are "going back [to hormones] because once the dust settles, more and more women and their doctors are beginning to understand that the risks of taking hormones are real but small indeed. "

Anecdotal commentary and clichés were pervasive in this report. The reporter deflected the scientific results of the WHI study with platitudes (e.g., "once the dust settles," "the baby [hormones] should not be thrown out with the bath water"). What could have been a serious, scientific discussion of the WHI results became superficial commentary and biased reporting. Unsubstantiated claims were made without explanation or discussion. The reporter commented, "For years the issue seemed black and white: women should take hormones as a sure way to stay healthy; few disputed these absolutes." This statement is inaccurate because in the last thirty years professional journals have presented different perspectives and ongoing debate about HRT: conflicting studies, editorials, dissenting letters, and opposing medical perspectives. Television talk shows have presented intense discussions with experts and women polarized. Never has there been an absolute consensus on the effectiveness or safety of HRT.

Many books have been written about hormone replacement therapy, menopause and aging. Although these books attempt to help women gain a better understanding of HRT, female biology and aging, they are often inadequate sources of information. Data is often presented selectively and out of context, making it difficult for the reader to evaluate the author's spin on the research. Lay books are frequently written by doctors who are biased for or against HRT. Since physicians are part of the medical establishment, they are usually entrenched in the current treatment paradigm or influenced by the pharmaceutical industry. Some books about HRT also patronize women by oversimplifying the information, giving insubstantial explanations and providing inadequate citations or no citations at all. Lacking focus, covering too many health topics superficially and failing to discuss cross-cultural ideas of approaches to aging and menopause, lay books on HRT often leave women with many questions but few answers.

This reference guide was written to address the inadequacies and biases about HRT presented in advertisements, television pieces and lay books. Written for women and their health care providers, it provides thorough citation and references, encouraging women to ask informed questions and to make science-based decisions about HRT. This guide reports the findings of both large and small clinical, case-control and cohort studies that have been peer reviewed and published in medical and scientific journals. For these studies to be accepted by the journals, the researchers had to follow specific ethical guidelines concerning their study populations, and their methodologies, data and sources were carefully scrutinized. Hence the studies represent a high level of professionalism and credibility.

This reference guide presents studies about HRT in a reader friendly style. It summarizes major findings, defines terms and keeps statistics to a minimum. Each study is organized into the following sections: Researchers/Authors, title of study, publication data, Type of Study, Focus of Study, Conclusions, Findings, Researchers' Comments, and Participants and Methods. The studies are arranged alphabetically by authors and presented by topic: Breast Cancer, Cardiovascular Conditions, Endometrial Cancer, Osteoporosis, Ovarian Cancer, and Other Conditions. An introduction discusses the questions about hormone replacement therapy. The section titled "Understanding Research Studies" explains the types of studies, how to interpret the data, and how to evaluate the research. In the back of the book, a glossary and a bibliography are provided to aid the reader with vocabulary, referencing and cross-referencing. The studies span 1970 through 2002.

Understanding menopause and health issues can help women make informed decisions about HRT. Answering some questions about hormone replacement therapy can help women clarify their health care choices and support better decision making: How do I feel about taking HRT for the short term or for life? Am I willing to accept the risks associated with HRT? What are my risk factors for certain diseases that may afflict aging women? How do women in other cultures deal with aging and menopause? Have I

explored other therapies (conventional or alternative) to deal with menopause and aging? Are my sources of information about HRT accurate and
unbiased? Women who examine the research will draw different conclusions concerning the risks and benefits of HRT based on their physiology,
risk factors and health perspectives.

Introduction

Women want information about health issues. Too often, however, advertisements or short discussions with a health care provider are their only sources of information about hormone replacement therapy (HRT). This reference guide presents research in a condensed and intelligible format to help women, with the support of their heath care providers, make informed decisions about HRT. Physiology, risk factors and health perspectives vary, and so will individual decisions.

Long-term HRT: Side Effects and Risks?

HRT can be used short-term to deal with menopausal symptoms such as hot flashes and insomnia; however, controversy surrounds the long-term use of HRT as preventive therapy. Estrogen (sometimes spelled oestrogen) is not benign. In December 2001, a federal panel recommended adding estrogen to the nation's list of cancer causing agents. Long-term use of estrogen or estrogen plus progestin has been associated with an increase in a women's risk of breast cancer, embolism, triglycerides, gall bladder disease, endometrial cancer and possibly ovarian cancer. Women who receive HRT require medical monitoring because of the associated risks. Two important clinical trials have provided and will continue to provide valuable data on the risks and benefits of HRT: the Women's Health Initiative and the Women's International Study of Long Duration Oestrogen after Menopause. The latter study is being conducted in 14 countries and will report results in 2012. The Women's Health Initiative, with 16,600 women, announced in July 2002 that they would end one arm of the study because

1

of alarming results: women who received combined therapy (estrogen plus progestin) after five years had an increased risk of heart attack (29 percent), stroke (41 percent) and breast cancer (26 percent).

Different Therapies, Different Results

Hormone replacement therapies (estrogen alone or combined therapy) may have different long-term effects. To complicate matters, the way HRT is ingested (e.g., transdermal or oral), the dosage given and the regimen (e.g., sequential vs. continuous) may have an impact on the long-term risks and benefits. As Dr. Susan Love argues, "We can't simply extrapolate the date from cyclical estrogen and progestin therapy to continuous therapy. Continuous progestins have a different effect on the heart than cyclical progestins, which means that they might have different effects in many other areas" (132).

Risk Factors for Diseases Vary Among Women

A woman's decision to use HRT includes an evaluation of her risk factors for various conditions that can influence longevity and quality of life (e.g., heart disease, osteoporosis, vascular conditions, breast cancer). For some women, even with common risk factors, their life expectancy will be different. Individual physiology, genetics and lifestyle affect life expectancy. The results of the important ongoing clinical trials and basic research about disease mechanisms may provide more definitive information.

Pharmaceutical, Dietary, and Supplement Treatments for Managing Hot Flashes and Other Symptoms

HRT is prescribed for the treatment of menopausal symptoms (hot flashes, insomnia, mood swings). However, other treatments for menopausal symptoms are available that do not have risks associated with HRT. Pharmaceutical alternatives to HRT to manage hot flashes include Effexor (an antidepressant), Clondine (blood pressure medicine), Aldomet (blood pressure medicine) and Bellergal (combination of three medications). One study found that hot flashes were reduced by 60 percent in women who used Effexor (Gottleb, 2000).

Dietary measures, herbs, homeopathic remedies and supplements have been used to treat menopausal symptoms. Some women have found relief from hot flashes by consuming soy products or flaxseed and reducing caffeine and alcohol consumption (Ojeda, 1995). Soy products contain an important isoflavone (genistein) which functions as an antiestrogen in some tissue and as a weak estrogen in others. Epidemiologic studies have found that cultures that consume soy-based foods have fewer menopausal symptoms, lower cancer risk and lower heart disease risks (Anderson et al., 1995; Messina et al., 1993; Wilcox et al., 1991). Researchers have also found that people who consume soy products have lower cholesterol (Sirtori et al., 1999; Gaddi et al., 1991). The isoflavones in soy can block angiogenesis (blood vessel formation) in tumor cells, stopping their invasion of cells. Soy contains important protease inhibitors that block the enzymes used by tumors to grow and migrate (Hann, 1998; Hass, 1997; Schneeman, 1996). Some researchers argue that the data is inconclusive regarding the benefits, risks and physiological effects of soy, especially for soy supplements (Ginsburg, 2000). Long-term clinical trials are needed to decide the effects of the active ingredients in soy products. Although for thousands of years, Asian women have consumed soy foods without adverse side effects, soy supplements may have a different effect than soy foods.

Dietary supplements that may reduce hot flashes and other menopausal symptoms include vitamin E (400–800 IU/daily) and herbs. Chinese and Western herbs used to treat hot flashes include licorice root, chaste berry, black cohosh, dong quai, fennel, wild yam root and motherwort. Natural progesterone as a cream has been used to reduce menopausal symptoms. Like pharmaceutical treatments, these alternative therapies should be evaluated in clinical trials for efficacy and safety. Women need to know that assumptions regarding the effectiveness of many alternative therapies are currently based on mostly anecdotal evidence, not controlled studies.

Health and Decision Making

Whatever health program a woman follows to manage menopause and aging, she can continue to educate herself and reevaluate her choices periodically with the support of her health care provider. Obtaining knowledge and understanding of the health issues surrounding aging and menopause will give her the foundation for making intelligent decisions about HRT and other health issues. This will involve evaluating risks, values, research, controversies and the alternatives. As Dr. Susan Love has noted, "It's a complicated business, and not all the answers are in yet" (Love, 1997).

Understanding Research Studies

Terms in *italics* are defined in the glossary.

This reference guide presents observational, experimental (clinical trials) and statistical studies on the topic of hormone replacement therapy. To understand and interpret the HRT research, a reader needs a general understanding of these different research approaches, their advantages and their disadvantages.

Observational Studies

Observational studies gather data on the occurrence of a disease in people under their normal life conditions. When selecting a study population (people who participate as subjects), researchers look for people who have been exposed to a factor thought to influence or inhibit the development of disease, and for people (for comparison) who have not been exposed to that factor. A *factor* might be a medication, a hormone, a chemical, a food, alcohol, cigarettes, or something in the person's environment. The study population is observed and monitored for the development of disease or other conditions.

Two observational approaches are *cohort studies* and *case-control studies*. The major difference between these two approaches is that cohort studies use participants who are initially free of the disease, while in case-control studies some participants have already developed the disease. Both methods allow researchers to estimate how exposure to one or more factors affects the risk of developing the disease.

The selection of the study design depends on current information about a disease, its *incidence* and its *latency period*. For example, if a disease is rare or has a long latency period, the case-control approach is useful because some of the people being studied have already developed the disease. Because the time between exposure to a factor and the development of a disease can be long, cohort studies are less suitable for a disease with long latency period or for the study of rare diseases.

Cohort Studies

A cohort study investigates a selected group of people prospectively— that is, with the expectation that some of them may develop a certain disease. Participants are assessed for exposure and nonexposure to a given factor (e.g., hormone use), then observed over time to see if any of the individuals develop the disease. Cohort studies are prospective because they follow participants forward in time after the beginning of the investigation. After researchers select the cohort (the group of people to be studied), they gather exposure data and general information such as occupation, medical status and socioeconomic data from the participants' medical records, interviews and questionnaires. Both the exposed and the unexposed study groups must be free of the disease under investigation at the beginning of a cohort study.

Investigators monitor and assess the participants periodically for general health and for the development of the disease. The frequency of examination and the duration of the follow-up period depends on the type of exposure and the outcome under investigation. Investigators gather data on disease outcomes from participants' hospital records, medical records, interviews, self reports and death certificates.

ADVANTAGES OF COHORT STUDIES

Cohort studies have advantages. Participants do not have to recall information that could be subject to human error, so the approach is less susceptible to bias. Because the exposure occurs before the development of the disease, there is also less potential for bias in assessing exposure. Neither the researcher nor the participant is prejudiced by previous knowledge of who has the disease and who does not. Incidence, new cases of the disease, can be identified in cohort studies allowing investigators to derive a *relative risk* for the disease under study. Because cohort studies are prospective, the time sequence between exposure and outcome of a disease can be more accurately determined than in other research designs. Lastly, multiple disease outcomes can be studied with this research design.

DISADVANTAGE OF COHORT STUDIES

Cohort studies have disadvantages. They require a very large study population, particularly if the disease has a low incidence. The larger the number of factors under study, the larger the cohort requirement. Cohort studies also require a long follow-up period, which is not only costly but causes attrition (loss of study subjects). Participants need to return at regular intervals to be examined for development of the disease, but instead they may drop out from a lack of interest, or they may move or die during the study. High attrition rates can weaken a study's validity and conclusions. Furthermore, other problems arise from changes in the status of the subjects. A change in residence, occupation or smoking habits may cause errors in classification of a subject's exposure. Lastly, cohort studies can be problematic over time because of changes in diagnostic criteria and in methodology affecting the classification of individuals.

Case-Control Studies

Case-control studies select people who have a disease (these people are called cases) and compare them with people who do not have the disease (these people are called controls). Characteristics of the study population or exposures to factors thought to play a role in the development of disease are the basis of comparison between cases and controls. This method is retrospective because it considers the possible influence of some past exposure, such as smoking or oral contraceptive use, to a person's present health. Rather than waiting years for the disease to develop, investigators gather data from the past to discover factors that might have caused the disease under study. Controls and cases are matched according to age, socioeconomic status, sex, diet, alcohol consumption, smoking, age, ethnicity and residency. Controls are frequently selected from the same institutions from which cases are selected. Hospital patients are often controls because they are easily identified and their records are readily accessible. Hospital controls are usually willing to participate in research and may have better recall of events. A problem with hospital controls is that they have health problems that may change study results. Because of the possibility of bias, some studies select controls from the general population. Community members such as neighbors and co-workers are often used as controls.

ADVANTAGES OF CASE-CONTROL STUDIES

Case-control studies are less expensive than cohort studies. They require fewer subjects and provide quicker results. Retrospective studies are appropriate for studying rare diseases and those diseases with long latency because the investigators do not have to wait for the disease to develop. Moreover, because they already have a population of cases, case-control studies can use a smaller sample than a cohort study to obtain information about the risk of developing a rare disease. In contrast, cohort studies need lengthy, large study populations to get data on the development of a rare disease and require time for the disease to develop in the study population. Unlike prospective studies, case-control studies do not require volunteers and do not have attrition problems because the information is gathered retrospectively (from past records) and derived from existing cases. Also, the study does not expose the participants to any factors—they have already been exposed to the medication or condition before the study—so there are no risks to the study subjects. Lastly, case-control studies can examine multiple exposure factors for a disease or condition.

DISADVANTAGES OF CASE-CONTROL STUDIES

Case-control studies have disadvantages. Information about past events may not be available from routine records or may be inaccurately recorded. Biased or selective recall can occur because participants or physicians may have inadequate information about an event or events in the past. Investigators may be more likely to search for explanation for the disease in the cases, and this could cause the interviewer unconsciously to scrutinize cases more closely. The more severe a disease, the more likely this kind of bias will occur. Problems selecting a control group can occur because hospitals or clinical rosters can be sources of bias if controls and cases are not carefully matched or are not similar to the general population. Cases may not include all those affected by the disease: hospitalized cases may exclude mild cases and those who die before admission. Because of this potential bias, a true association between a factor and the development of disease may be masked or misinterpreted. Another disadvantage of case-control studies is that because the incidence (number of new disease cases) cannot be known but only estimated, therefore the relative risk can only be estimated. In case-control studies, researches use a statistic called the *odds ratio* to approximate the relative risk. Case-control studies are sometimes criticized because the odds ratio overestimates or underestimates the relative risk (Zhang & Yu, 1998).

Experimental Studies

Researchers employ two experimental approaches: animal studies and human clinical trials. In both approaches, the investigator studies the impact of varying some factor that is under his or her control. Animal experiments occur in a laboratory setting, and human clinical trials usually occur in hospitals or clinics. When humans are used to study a disease, drug or treatment, the process involves initiating a clinical trial.

For a clinical trial, researchers select consenting individuals with similar risk factors and socioeconomic characteristics. The participants are then randomly assigned to one of two groups, a treatment group and a placebo or control group (no treatment). Random allocation to a group eliminates any bias that would result if the researcher or participant chose the group. The study group is exposed to a factor or treatment—for example, HRT or heart medication. Then the two groups are observed and monitored for the development of the disease or condition under study.

Human clinical trials use a method called blinding to eliminate potential bias. Most clinical trials are double blinded: neither the researcher nor the participants know to which group the participants are assigned. This is important because the expectations of the researcher or participant can produce bias in a study. Double blinded studies are particularly important in research where subjective endpoints (e.g., improved, unchanged, worse) are used.

Advantages of the Experimental Approach

Many researchers and physicians consider the experimental approach to be the gold standard of research. The experimental approach can help establish the causes and effects of disease more conclusively than observational studies. With this method, the investigators follow the effects of a factor over time by carefully controlling who receives treatment and who does not. If an exposed group in a trial develops more disease than the unexposed group (placebo group), there is strong evidence that the factor does increase risk of the disease; subsequent studies should confirm this finding. Usually, clinical trials involve preventing disease (prophylactic trials) or treating an existing disease (therapeutic trials). The strengths of the experimental approach—random allocation, placebo and study groups, and the double-blind technique—remove the effects of *confounding variables* that can alter or distort the outcome of the research.

Disadvantages of
the Experimental Approach

The experimental approach has disadvantages. It requires a lengthy study period and demands meticulous study methods. Long studies, such as those that focus on agents thought to prevent cancer, can take up to twenty years because of the long latency between exposure to a carcinogen and the development of the disease. Long, extensive studies are expensive and resource intensive which often results in economic problems and attrition. Nonparticipation and attrition can lead to results that may be flawed and misinterpreted. Worse, the results from the trial might be wrongly applied to the general population.

Study methods such as blinding and randomization are sometimes misused. Many published, randomized controlled trials have not been double-blinded. Blinding in some studies may be ineffective because of poor explanations or methods used for double blinding. For example, researchers may not report excluded patients in their published papers.

Another problem resulting from a long study period is that medical technologies change. Sometimes a method under investigation in a clinical trial may have become obsolete by the time the trial is completed. An example of this would be a ten-year investigation of a surgical approach that becomes outdated because of rapid technological changes in the field.

Clinical trials may also involve ethical questions that provoke controversy, especially if treatment has risks for the participants or if withholding treatment from a placebo group has adverse health consequences. Other ethical issues also involve the use of animals in experimental research. People for the Ethical Treatment of Animals (PETA) has publicized the animal rights issues and criticized animal studies. According to PETA, results from animal studies are not applicable to humans because animals have their own unique physiology and respond differently to medication than people do.

Statistical Studies (Meta-analysis)

Meta-analysis is a statistical approach to synthesizing and analyzing data. Meta-analysis compares the relative risk or odds ratio from multiple studies, then computes an average risk. Employing systematic rules, meta-analysis includes a detailed description of the study methods, making it easier for the reader to interpret the research. This approach can yield more statistical power, but it cannot eliminate the weaknesses and biases of individual studies.

Advantages and Disadvantages
of Meta-analysis

This method is less subjective than a narrative review that can reflect bias in the author's selection of studies discussed. However, combining data from individual studies into an average diminishes the meaning that individual studies convey. Reliance on quantitative information may cloud understanding with a barrage of numbers and data. Combining data from many studies has the potential for problems if the studies have different populations and dissimilar research designs. Investigators using a meta-analysis must be careful in the selection of studies to avoid biased conclusions. Lastly, if the data from those studies is inaccurate, the result from the meta-analysis may distort and misrepresent the problems under investigation.

Interpreting and Evaluating the Research

Relative Risk and Odds Ratio

Observational and experimental studies measure risk using relative risk or odds ratio. Relative risk is used in cohort studies and clinical trials. Relative risk compares the incidence rate of a disease in two groups, one exposed to a given factor and the other unexposed. Thus, investigators compare the risks of two different groups. Researchers look for association between exposure to a factor and development of a disease or condition. To this association they assign a numerical value. The further the relative risk from the value of 1.00 (no association), the stronger the association and the more likely a cause and effect relationship exists between exposure to the factor and the development of a disease. A relative risk of less than 1.00 suggests that there is less risk in the exposed group than in the non-exposed group. The larger the relative risk, the less likely the association is due to chance. For example, if the risk of developing breast cancer is 3.00 for hormone users after ten years of hormone use and 1.00 for nonusers, then hormone users will have three times the risk of developing breast cancer than nonusers. Examining relative risk in the context of rare diseases or conditions is important. Sometimes even with an increased relative risk for a condition, a person with an exposure factor would not have a very high probability of developing a disease or condition that has a low incidence and *prevalence*. For example, as some researchers have noted, "women who have used oral contraceptives for a long time have a high relative risk of developing liver cell adenoma. However, the underlying incidence of the disease is so small that the increased risk assumed by the users is insignificant in comparison to the benefits gained" (Morton & Hebel, 34). Thus a higher risk for a rare disease may be of less concern than a moderate risk for a disease with a higher incidence. Age is also important when considering risk. For example, the risk of breast cancer increases as a woman ages regardless of her existing risk factors for the disease.

Odds ratio, a measure of risk used in case-control studies, compares the odds of disease in a group exposed to a factor with the odds of disease in a group not exposed to a factor. Case-control studies obtain data from the past, so they cannot determine relative risk that is based on incidences (new cases of disease). Instead, case-control studies estimate relative risk using the odds ratio. For the odds ratio to be an acceptable measure of risk, the disease in question must have a low incidence in the general population.

Measures of risk are statements of probability, not absolute predictions of future outcomes. Statistical associations do not explain or prove causation. Not all individuals exposed to a factor develop disease, and some who have not been exposed to a factor develop disease. Some diseases are thought to be caused by multiple factors. If a statistical *association* makes physiological sense, a researcher may form a *hypothesis* (theory) about cause and effect that future studies will either support or negate.

Study Size, Confounding Variables and Selection Bias

Complex scientific information is often open to varied interpretation. Individuals will bring different perspectives and values to a problem. Examination of prior information is an important part of scientific evaluation because a body of information, not just one study, forms the basis of theories about disease, risks and causation. Studies should be examined within the context of earlier research. The results of a recent study do not necessarily override the conclusions of an earlier study. If a recent study has a poor design—weak controls, population bias, small sample size, confounding factors—the results from earlier research may in fact be more valid and reliable.

Instead of providing answers, studies often raise more questions. More data may need to be collected, and long-term clinical trials may be required to sort out contradictory results, answer questions and eliminate confounding factors. Research design is important when evaluating the studies, particularly the size of the study. Larger studies have greater statistical power, validity (accuracy) and reliability. The greater the number of cases, the more probable the conclusion. For example, if two treatments are being studied, a large clinical trial would be necessary to yield a small margin of error. The smaller a study, the more likely the results are a product of chance. Furthermore, if the effect of a treatment is small yet important, only a large study will reveal the significance.

The methods used to compile and interpret data and the characteristics of the study population affect research results. Errors in and omissions of data alter the results of studies and lead to dubious conclusions. Confounding variables are factors that need to be accounted for because they can affect results. For example, in one study the effects of HRT (combined therapy) and Simvastatin were evaluated in postmenopausal women with elevated cholesterol. The original investigators reported 27 percent reduction in Lp(a) lipoprotein levels in women using HRT (Darling et al., 1997). Other researchers (Cashen-Hemphill et al., 1998) criticized the conclusions of the study, arguing that the researchers did not consider the effects of dietary changes on lipoproteins and needed to document dietary composition at base line and during treatment. These researchers noted the problem of not controlling for an important variable such as diet and its impact on the results of the study.

Selection bias involves an unrepresentative study population—unrepresentative in either health or economic status—that can distort the results of a study. The "healthy user effect" is an example of selection bias where the study population is healthier than the general population. It has been identified as a problem in some HRT studies. Some researchers have argued that the lower incidence of heart disease and better cholesterol levels found in estrogen users may be a result of a population of study subjects that are healthier and receive more consistent monitoring and health care (Derby et al., 1995). Women who receive HRT are mostly Caucasian, lean, diet conscious, educated and upper-middle class. They may have healthy lifestyles and access to health care that other women do not have. As one health expert has argued, "Women getting hormones have been at low risk for heart disease and breast cancer to start with. This selection bias—studying women at low risk to start with—means that all observational studies are likely to end up overestimating any benefits in terms of controlling heart disease and underestimating the dangers in terms of contributing to breast cancer" (Love, 1997, p. 68).

Questions to Ask to Evaluate the Research

The following questions are important to consider when one examines research studies. These questions can aid the reader in evaluating the research:

- Does the study support or contradict previous findings?
- Does the study need verification with future research (e.g., a clinical trial)?
- Does the study present some important new data or protocol?
- Does the study employ sound research methods (e.g., size, statistics, design, population selection, controls)?
- Is the study randomized and/or double blind?
- Are the *endpoints* or outcomes clearly and objectively defined (e.g., survival rate, quality of life)?
- Was use of medications explained (type, dosage and duration of use)?
- Were the confounding factors considered and were they adjusted for?
- Could other variables have accounted for the results of the study?
- In cohort studies, was the follow-up explained?
- In cohort studies and clinical trials, were all outcomes (e.g., breast cancer) compared in exposed and comparison groups?
- Who funded the study, what is the relationship of the researchers to the funding institution, and is there a potential conflict of interest?

1

Breast Cancer

Breast cancer involves the abnormal growth and proliferation of cells in breast tissues. It usually starts in the lining of the milk ducts as a pre-cancerous condition (DCIS, *ductal carcinoma in situ*). If these cells leave the ducts and invade other tissue, metastasis occurs when the breast cancer cells invade the blood vessels and spread to other organs. Other than skin cancer, breast cancer is the most common type of cancer in women in the United States. Breast cancer incidence had changed liitle during the 1990s, but breast cancer death rates have declined about 2 percent per year since 1990 and have decreased since 1995. Based on cancer rates from 1997 through 1999, the National Cancer Institute estimated that a woman has a 1 in 8 chance of being diagnosed with breast cancer in her lifetime. The average age for breast cancer is 69 years. The risk and incidence for breast cancer increases with age: approximately 1 woman in 252 for age 30–40 years, 1 woman in 35 for age 50–60 years, 1 woman in 27 for age 60–70 years. Caucasian, Hawaiian and black women have the highest risk of developing breast cancer. Women with more risk factors are also at increased risk for breast cancer, but 70 percent of breast cancer cases are women with no known risk factors. Only 5 to 10 percent of breast cancer cases result from genetics, BRCA1 or BRCA2 genes (http://www.seer.cancer.gov; http://www.meds.com).

The Etiology of Breast Cancer Is Uncertain

The development of breast cancer probably involves the interplay of environmental exposures and a propensity to develop the disease. Explanations of and theories about risks of developing breast cancer are less con-clusive than those of heart disease: the data is more conflicting and envi-ronmental causes are less clear-cut. For example, a diet high in saturated fat is definitely associated with an increased risk of heart disease. This relationship has been documented in many studies on heart disease. With breast cancer, the relationship between diet and the disease is still an enigma. Some studies have found a relationship between diet and the devel-opment of breast cancer (Jardin et al, 2002); others have not found any relationship (Willete et al., 1987). Alcohol consumption may benefit the heart, but not the breasts (Hamajima et al., 2002; Singletary & Gapstur, 2001). Alcohol consumption increases circulating estrogen levels and in higher amounts can significantly elevate estrogen levels. Women who use HRT and drink alcohol have a pronounced increase of 22 percent in blood estradiol levels (Ginsburg et al., 1996). Possible etiologies of breast cancer include reproductive, hormonal, genetic, environmental and familial fac-tors. Risk factors that may contribute to the development of breast cancer are a family history of breast cancer, abnormal breast biopsies and breast cysts, lifetime exposure to estrogen and progesterone (endogenous sources and HRT), lack of exercise, exposure to chemicals that mimic estrogens (e.g., pesticides, organochlorines, dioxins) use of alcohol and tobacco, con-sumption of high fat diet or diets low in fruits and vegetables, obesity, early menarche and late menopause, first pregnancy after age thirty, infertility due to lack of ovulation, nulliparity, longterm use of combination oral con-traceptives starting at a young age or use of the injectable contraceptive—depot-medroxyprogesterone acetate (DMPA/Depo-Provera) and exposure to ionizing radiation.

HRT and Breast Cancer

Hormone replacement therapy has been associated with an increased risk of breast cancer in many but not all observational and clinical trials dating from the early 1970s to the present. Comparing the results of the studies can be difficult because of differences in study populations, method-ologies, types of HRT and dosages and duration of therapies (Steinberg et al., 1991). Many earlier studies used higher dosages of estrogen (0.625–1.25 mg/d) and evaluated estrogen alone therapy not combined therapy. How-ever, more recent studies that have evaluated combined therapy (estrogen + progestin) also found an increased risk of breast cancer in women who received HRT (Colditz et al., 1995; WHI Writing Group, 2002; Chen et al., 2002). Some research shows a dose response relationship with those women who receive higher doses of estrogen having a greater risk; whereas, some studies have found the risk of developing breast cancer more dependent on the duration of estrogen use (Steinberg et al., 1991). Although the biological mechanism for estrogen's role in the development of breast cancer is not totally understood, it is known that estrogen is a tumor promotor, causing tumor cells to proliferate in vitro. Also, breast cancer cells that have estrogen-positive receptors are fueled by exposure to estrogen. Research has also shown that antiestrogens, such as raloxifene block estrogen receptors on cells so estrogen cannot stimulate growth (Kennedy 1995; Lamartiniere 1995; Cummings et al., 1999).

Preventing Breast Cancer

Since the etiology of breast cancer is uncertain, preventing breast cancer is about making the lifestyle choices with the best current knowledge and technology. Preventative measures can involve regular screening, genetic testing for high risk women, use of antiestrogens, eating an antioxidant-rich diet and living a healthy lifestyle. Although not perfect tools, mammography, self-exams and ultrasound can be used to help detect breast cancer in its early stages. Studies regarding the benefits of mammography are conflicting and controversy surrounds the issue of screening women in their forties. However, for women over fifty, the benefits of mammography are more substantial with reduced mortality from the disease. Women over fifty have more fatty breast tissue, allowing mammography to identify tumors more accurately, whereas younger women have denser breast tissue making tumors hard to detect with mammography. Estrogen therapy increases breast density and reduces the sensitivity and accuracy of mammography (Laya et al., 1996). Genetic testing can inform a woman if she carries a genetic propensity for breast cancer (e.g., mutated BRCA genes). Antiestrogens, such as tamoxifen and raloxifene have been given to women at high risk for developing breast cancer or who have had breast cancer. Tamoxifen and adjuvant therapy for early stage breast cancer reduces the risk of recurrence of the disease by 50 percent (http://www.cancer.gov). Eating a diet rich in fruits and vegetables, obtaining consistent exercise, avoiding environmental toxins, limiting exposure to radiation, carefully evaluating hormone use, breast-feeding children, maintaining a healthy weight, avoiding smoking and controlling alcohol consumption may be sensible approaches to lowering a woman's risk of the disease. Many questions about the disease need to be answered through trials and basic research. Research is under way to develop more sensitive diagnostic tests such as blood tests that may identify proteins in women who have breast cancer.

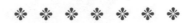

➤ **Bergkvist L, Adami H-O, Persson I, Hoover R, and Schairer C.**

The risk of breast cancer after estrogen and estrogen-progestin replacement. *The New England Journal of Medicine*, August 1989; 321:293–297. **Type:** Observational (cohort)

Focus: An analysis of the risk of *breast cancer* after treatment with estrogen and combined therapy (*estrogen + progestin*).

Conclusions: An increased risk of breast cancer was found in women who received HRT. The risk increased with increasing duration of HRT use. The risk of breast cancer was highest among women who used combined therapy (estrogen + progestin) for long periods. The addition of progestin did not reduce the risk and may actually increase the risk of breast cancer.

Findings:
• A higher risk of breast cancer was associated with longer duration of estrogen treatment.
• No association was found between weaker estrogens (mainly *estriol*) and the development of breast cancer, but there was an association with the use of stronger estrogen such as estradiol.
• An elevated risk of breast cancer was found with the use of *estradiol*, particularly in women who had used HRT for six to nine years (***relative risk:*** 2.30 for users/1.00 for nonusers).
• A 30 percent increase in risk of breast cancer was found in women who used *conjugated estrogens* for six or more years.
• The addition of progestin did not protect against the development of breast cancer.

Researchers' Comments: "In the US studies, a conjugated estrogen dose of 1.25 mg or more was most common whereas in our cohort most women used only 0.625 mg" (296).

Participants and Methods: The cohort consisted of 23,244 women (35 years or older) from Sweden who had estrogen prescriptions filled. The researchers evaluated the risk of breast cancer for different types of estrogen used and the use of progestin. The study began in April 1977 and ended in 1980. The follow-up (about 6 years) of the development of breast cancer was done by linking the National registration number of these women with those of the newly diagnosed breast cancer reported to the National Cancer Registry in Sweden. The investigators identified 253 cases of breast cancer. A subgroup, which was selected randomly from the 23,444 cohorts of women, was used to characterize the women more accurately about HRT use and risk factors for breast cancer. Questionnaires were sent to this group to obtain data in 1980, 1982 and 1984.

➤ **Bland K, Buchanan J, Weisberg B, Hagan T, and Gray L.**

The effects of exogenous estrogen replacement therapy of the breast cancer risk and mammographic parenchymal pattern. *Cancer*, June 1980; 45:3027–3033. **Type:** Observational (case-control)

Focus: An examination of the effects of HRT and its relationship to breast tissue and breast cancer.

Conclusions: Long-term HRT does not significantly alter breast tissue, nor does HRT increase the risk of breast cancer.

Findings:

• The risk of cancer was not higher in any category in relation to HRT use.
• A higher frequency in the occurrence of breast cancer was observed in women who were nonusers of HRT.
• A lower frequency of breast cancer was observed in users of HRT.
• No association was found with the use of HRT and the development of breast cancer.

Researchers' Comments: "Endocrine regulation of breast growth and neoplasia is complex and involves many hormones including estrogen and progesterone, growth hormone, prolactin, thyroxin and adrenal steroids.... [A]dministration of these conjugated compounds on a cyclic basis may have a potential neoplastic role" (3027).

Participants and Methods: The sources of the data for this study were the records and case histories of 14,023 female patients from the Louisville Breast Cancer Detection Demonstration Project, the Breast Diagnostic Center, or the office practice of one of the authors. Patients were classified as having symptomatic breast disease or being asymptomatic. Four-hundred and five women were identified, analyzed and compared. All participants were assessed for general health, medical conditions, medications and estrogen use. Fifty-four symptomatic women were identified as long-term HRT users. These women were matched with nonusers according to age and *parity*. Mammographic information was obtained for all the participants.

➤ **Brinton L, Hoover R, Szklo M, and Fraumeni J.**

Menopausal estrogens use and risk of breast cancer. *Cancer,* May 1981; 47:2517–2522. **Type:** Observational (case-control)

Focus: An assessment of the relationship of menopausal estrogens to breast cancer risk.

Conclusions: Estrogen use may increase the risk of breast cancer. The risk was highest in women who had *oophorectomies* and were long term users of HRT. Long term and high dosage HRT were associated with an elevated risk of breast cancer.

Findings:

• A 70 percent increased risk of breast cancer was observed in women who had used HRT for 10 or more years (*relative risk estimate:* 1.70 for users/1.00 for nonusers).

• No consistent findings were related to age at first birth, age at *menopause* or age at first use of HRT.

• Among women who had been oophorectomized, the highest risk of breast cancer was observed in women who had other risk factors: *nulliparity*, maternal history of breast cancer, a history of a previous breast biopsy.

• Higher dose estrogen therapy was associated with increased risk of breast cancer.

Researchers' Comments: "This case-control study revealed the complexities of evaluating the relationship between menopausal hormone use and risk of breast cancer" (2520).

Participants and Methods: The women in this study were selected from a multicenter screening program, the Breast Cancer Detection Demonstration Project. This program recruited about 280,000 women age 35–74 years from 29 centers across the United States for annual screening over a five-year period. The screening consisted of physical examination, mammography and thermography. The cases were women who were diagnosed with breast cancer between July 1973 and May 1977. These women were matched with controls for the following factors: breast detection center, race, age (within five years) and duration of participation in the screening program.

➤ **Burch J and Byrd B.**

Effects of long-term administration of estrogen on the occurrence of mammary cancer in women. **Annals of Surgery**, September 1971; 174: 414–418. **Type:** Observational (cohort)

Focus: An investigation of the relationship between long-term HRT and the occurrence of breast cancer in women who had *hysterectomies*.

Conclusions: Long-term use of HRT did not increase the incidence of breast cancer. Mortality rates declined in long-term HRT users who had hysterectomies.

Findings:

• No increase in breast cancer was found in women who had hysterectomies and who had used HRT (mostly conjugated estrogen) long-term.

• A delay in the onset of breast cancer was observed in HRT users who had hysterectomies.

• The incidence of breast cancer in the study group was similar to nonusers of the same group.

Researchers' Comments: "On the basis of our study, the administration of estrogens is associated with a drop in the anticipated incidence of all cancers and particularly those other than malignancies of the breast" (418).

Participants and Methods: This cohort was 511 women (27 to 72 years) who had undergone hysterectomies and received HRT postoperatively (primarily conjugated estrogen). The subjects were followed postoperatively from approximately 1960 to determine the incidence of breast cancer, general mortality and mortality from cancer alone.

▶ **Burch J, Byrd B, and Vaughn W.**

The effects of long-term estrogen on hysterectomized women. *American Journal of Obstetrics and Gynecology*, March 1974; 118:778–782. **Type:** Observational (cohort)

Focus: An evaluation of the role of estrogen in the development of breast cancer.

Conclusions: No increased incidence of breast cancer or other cancers was found in women who used HRT. Low mortality rates were also observed in women who received HRT.

Findings:

• Women who had hysterectomies and used HRT had low mortality.

• Women who had hysterectomies and used HRT had a low incidence of all cancers.

• A delayed onset of osteoporosis was found in women who had hysterectomies and used HRT.

Researchers' Comments: "Obviously, estrogen is not the answer to all problems which beset the older woman and the final chapter has yet to be written with regard to its *prophylactic* value in the prevention of osteo-porosis, *atherosclerosis* or aging" (782).

Participants and Methods: A log of hysterectomies performed by one of the authors from the 1940's to 1967 was the basis of the study pool. Beginning in July 1973, the cohort included 737 women for a total of 9,869 patient years. The women in this study received HRT (conjugated estrogen) and were followed-up to see if death or disease developed.

> **Buring J, Hennekens C, Lipnick R, Willett W, Stampfer M, Rosner B, Peto R, and Speizer F.**

A prospective cohort study of postmenopausal women hormone use and risk of breast cancer in US women. *American Journal of Epidemiology*, June 1987; 125:939–947. **Type:** Observational (cohort)

Focus: An investigation of the risk of breast cancer in women receiving HRT.

Conclusions: Women who used HRT on a short-term basis (less than five years) did not have increased risk of breast cancer. However, long-term use may increase a woman's risk of breast cancer.

Findings:
• Neither current nor past use of HRT was associated with an increase in breast cancer risk.
• No increased risk of breast cancer was found in women who used HRT for five years or less.
• Women who used HRT for more than five years had a slight increased risk of breast cancer (**relative risk:** 1.50 for users/1.00 for nonusers).
• The type of menopause did not affect the risk of breast cancer in HRT users.

Reseachers' Comments: "If many years after postmenopausal hormone use a small increase in the incidence of breast cancer were to emerge, a sizable number of women would be affected, since currently one out of every 12 women in the United States will develop breast cancer" (946).

Participants and Methods: In 1976, the American Nurses' Association provided the names and addresses of all married, female registered nurses aged 30–55 years residing in the US. The participants, 121,964 post-menopausal women with no history of cancer, formed the cohort of the Nurses' Health Study. The women were sent questionnaires requesting information regarding health issues and medical history including an assessment of postmenopausal hormone use and breast cancer risks. Follow-up was conducted in 1978 and June 1980. The 1976 questionnaire did not include information on the type of hormone; however, the 1978 questionnaire included that item and indicated that the most commonly used HRT was conjugated. The effect of different dosages of postmenopausal hormones was not evaluated.

➤ Chen C-L, Weiss N, Newcomb P, Barlow W, and White E.

Hormone replacement therapy in relation to breast cancer. *Journal of the American Medical Association*, February 2002; 287:734–741.

Type: Observational (case-control)

Focus: An investigatiin of the association between HRT and the risk of breast cancer based on type of HRT and histology of cancer.

Conclusions: Long-term use of HRT is associated with an increased risk of breast cancer, especially lobular tumors.

Findings:

• Postmenopausal women who were long-term users (5 years or more) of oral estrogen, either alone or in combination with progestin had an increased risk of invasive breast cancer.

• A 60 percent to 85 percent increased risk of breast cancer was found in women who used oral estrogen alone, *combined therapy, sequential therapy* or *continuous therapy*.

• HRT was strongly associated with an increased risk of lobular breast cancer, with a particular high risk associated with long-term and current combined therapy (**odds ratio:** 3.91 for current users of combined therapy).

• Long-term use of HRT was associated with a 50 percent increased risk of nonlobular cancer.

• Past users of HRT did not have an increased risk of breast cancer.

Researchers' Comments: "A true increase in the risk of lobular breast cancer could have implications for screening, because lobular carcinomas are relatively more difficult to palpate and more difficult to diagnose by mammography" (740).

Participants and Methods: The cases, 705 women (50–74 years), were enrolled in the Group Health Cooperative of Puget Sound who were diagnosed with breast cancer between 1990 and 1995. The women were identified through the Seatle–Puget Sound Surveillance, Epidemiology, and End Results cancer registry. The controls, 692 women, were randomly selected from the enrollment files of GHC and were matched with cases by year and age of diagnosis and years of GHC enrollment. Information about reproductive history, estrogen use, family history of breast

cancer, mammography and other health issues was gathered from questionnaires.

➤ Cobleigh M, Norlock F, Oleske D, and Starr A.

Hormone replacement therapy and high S phase in breast cancer.
Journal of the American Medical Association, April 1999; 281:1528–
1530. **Type:** Observational (cohort)

Focus: A comparison of the type of breast cancers in women who
have received HRT and women who have never used HRT.

Conclusions: HRT is associated with *estrogen receptor positive* breast
cancer, but not *estrogen receptor negative* breast cancer.

Findings:
- Women who had received HRT (combined therapy or estrogen alone)
  had increased S-phase growth of cancer.
- Women who had used HRT had more estrogen receptor positive breast
  cancer than non-users (*relative risk:* 5.25 for users/1.00 for nonusers).
- Women who had used HRT did not have a significant higher rate of
  estrogen receptor negative breast cancer than nonusers (*relative
  risk:* 1.08 for users/1.00 for nonusers).
- Estrogen receptor positive cancers were affected by HRT: current users
  with ER-positve breast cancer were five times more likely to have high
  phase cancer growth.
- Users of HRT (combined therapy or estrogen alone) were 40.7 percent
  of the participants. Past users of HRT were 47.3 percent of the women
  and never users of HRT were 10.9 percent.

Researchers' Comments: "Estrogen causes proliferation of ER-
positive but not ER-negative human breast cancer cells *in vitro* and *in vivo*...."
(1529)

Participants and Methods: This cohort study, conducted from
1989 to 1996, recruited participants at a teaching hospital in a large Mid-
western urban area. The participants were 331 postmenopausal women with
invasive breast cancer. The women were assessed for general health, medical conditions, cancer characteristics (e.g., receptor type/percentage of cells
in S phage), medications, reproductive history and estrogen use.

➤ Colditz G, Stampher M, Willett W, Hennekens C, Rosner B, and Speizer F.

Prospective study of estrogen replacement therapy and risk of breast
cancer in postmenopausal women. *Journal of the American Medical*

Association, November 1990; 264:2648–2652. **Type:** Observational (cohort)

Focus: An investigation of the relationship between HRT and breast cancer incidences.

Conclusions: An elevated risk of breast cancer was found among current and recent past users of HRT. Women who currently used HRT had a higher risk of breast cancer than nonusers.

Findings:

• Current users of HRT were more likely to have a history of benign breast disease, to be lean and to consume alcohol.

• Current users of HRT were more inclined to have been nulliparious or to have given birth once or twice.

• An elevated risk of breast cancer associated with HRT increased with age (*relative risk:* 2.13 for current users aged 60–64 years/1.09 for past users aged 60–64 years).

• Current users of HRT had a greater risk of breast cancer than past users (*relative risk:* 1.40 for current users/0.99 for past users/1.00 for nonusers).

Researchers' Comments: "The prospective design of this study greatly reduces the possibility of bias due to the reporting of postmenopausal hormone use" (2651).

Participants and Methods: The data presented in this prospective study was derived from the ongoing Nurses' Health Study initiated in 1976. The study included 23,607 postmenopausal nurses (30–55 years old) who participated in follow-up from 1976 to 1978. These women had similar ages at menarche and similar family histories of breast cancer. Menopause status was updated every two years and the population was expanded to included women who became postmenopausal and who did not have cancer. At baseline the women were assessed for general health, medical conditions, breast cancer risk factors, menopausal status and HRT (type). Alcohol consumption and dose of estrogen were first recorded in 1980. Follow-up questionnaires have been mailed every two years to update the information. The end point for this study was the occurrence of breast cancer; consequently, any woman who reported breast cancer or other cancer (except non-melanoma skin cancer) on the 1976 questionnaire was excluded from this study.

➤ **Colditz G, Egan K, and Stampfer M.**

Hormone replacement therapy and risk of breast cancer: results from epidemiologic studies. *American Journal of Obstetrics and Gynecology*, May 1993; 168:1473–1479. **Type:** Statistical (meta-analysis)

Focus: An evaluation of combined data from published reports of the relation between HRT and the development of breast cancer.

Conclusions: Women who have used estrogen in the past, but have stopped for more than two years are not at an increased risk of breast cancer. However, current use may be related to an increased risk of developing breast cancer. Family history of breast cancer and personal history of benign breast disease do not affect the relationship between HRT and the development of breast cancer. Combined therapy (estrogen + progestin) does not reduce the risk of breast cancer.

Findings:

- The type of menopause did not affect the risk of breast cancer.
- Ever use of HRT was not associated with a significant increased risk of breast cancer.
- An increase in the risk of breast cancer was found in women who used HRT for ten or more years (*relative risk:* 1.23 for users/1.00 for nonusers).
- No association was found between different doses of HRT and the risk of breast cancer.
- A family history of breast cancer did not increase the risk of developing breast cancer among women who used HRT.
- Women who had used *diethylstilbestrol* had a 28 percent increased risk of breast cancer; women who had used combined therapy (estrogen + progestin) had a 13 percent increased risk of breast cancer, and women who had used conjugated estrogen had a 5 percent increased risk of breast cancer.

Researchers' Comments: "Although these results exclude a large effect of hormone therapy on breast cancer risk, we are unable to rule out some risk associated with current or long-term estrogen use" (1479).

Participants and Methods: The authors used MEDLINE to obtain information about HRT research. They pooled results separately from studies reporting HRT ever used, from studies reporting current use, or from studies using different HRT regimens.

➤ **Colditz G, Hankinson S, Hunter D, Willett C, Manson E, Stampfer M, Hennekens C, Rosner B, and Spiezer F.**

The use of estrogens and progestins and the risk of breast cancer. *The New England Journal of Medicine*, June 1995; 332:1589–1593. **Type:** Observational (cohort)

Focus: An investigation of the risk for breast cancer in postmenopausal women who used HRT.

Conclusions: The addition of progestins to estrogen therapy does not reduce the risk of breast cancer among postmenopausal women. Women with few risk factors for heart disease may not benefit from HRT, and estrogen therapy (short-term) may not protect postmenopausal women from fractures resulting from osteoporosis as they age. Combined therapy (estrogen + progestin) or estrogen alone is associated with a higher risk or developing breast cancer.

Findings:
- For each age at menopause the relative risk of breast cancer was equally high for women taking estrogen plus progestin or conjugated estrogen alone.
- The relative risk of breast cancer was highest among older women who were currently taking HRT, particularly those more than 55 years old.
- A significant increase in breast cancer was found in women who were currently using HRT for a period of five years or more. These women had an a 54 percent increased risk of breast cancer compared to nonusers (*relative risk:* 1.46 for users/1.00 for nonusers).
- No consistent risk of breast cancer was found for shorter duration of HRT.
- Women who had used HRT for five or more years and had discontinued therapy were at increased risk of breast cancer for only a short duration.
- Women who used conjugated estrogen alone had an increased risk for breast cancer compared to nonusers (*relative risk:* 1.32 for users/1.00 for nonusers).

Researchers' Comments: "The substantial increase in the risk of breast cancer among older women who take hormones suggests that the tradeoffs between risks and benefits be carefully assessed"(1589).

Participants and Methods: The data in this study is a result of a follow-up of the Nurses' Health Study which was implemented in 1976. Questionnaires were used to gather information from 121,700 nurses (30–55 years). Baseline information about the participants included general health, medical conditions, reproductive history, medications, risk factors for breast cancer and cardiovascular disease, use of oral contraceptives and postmenopausal use of hormones. Every two years a follow-up was performed: questionnaires were mailed updating information about menopausal status, hormone use and breast cancer status.

➤ **Cummings S, Eckert S, Krueger K, Grady D, Powles T, Cauley J, Norton L, Nickelsen T, Bjarnason N, Morrow M, Lippman M, Black D, Glusman J, Costa A, and Jordan C.**

The effect of raloxifene on risk of breast cancer in postmenopausal women: results from the MORE randomized trial. *Journal of the American Medical Association*, June 1999; 281:2189–2197. **Type:** Experimental (clinical trial)

Focus: An investigation to determine whether women receiving *raloxifene* for osteoporosis have a lower risk of invasive breast cancer.

Conclusions: Postmenopausal women using raloxifene for osteoporosis have a reduced risk of invasive, *estrogen receptor-positive breast cancer*, but no decrease in the risk of estrogen receptor-negative breast cancer.

Findings:

• 54 cases provided the data for this study: 13 cases of breast cancer occurred among the 5129 women who received raloxifene; 27 cases of breast cancer among 2576 women who received the placebo (**relative risk:** 0.24 for users/1.00 for nonusers).

• Raloxifene increased the risk of *thromboembolism* (**relative risk:** 3.10 for users/1.00 for nonusers).

• Women who used raloxifene did not have an increased risk of endometrial cancer (**relative risk:** 0.80 for users/1.00 for nonusers).

• More women in the raloxifene groups reported the onset or worsening of diabetes mellitus.

Researchers' Comments: "It is important to determine the long-term effects of raloxifene and other *selective estrogen receptor modulators* because metastatic breast cancer can develop resistance to tamoxifen after long-term exposure" (2195).

Participants and Methods: The Multiple Outcomes of Raloxifene Evaluation (MORE) study, conducted at 180 clinical centers in 25 countries, was double-blinded and lasting three years (1994–1998). Enrolled were 7705 postmenopausal women (96 percent Caucasian) with osteoporosis and an average age of 66.5 years. The women were assessed for general health, medical conditions, reproductive history, medications and estrogen use. Breast exams and mammography were also performed. Women were excluded for the following reasons: a history of breast cancer or other cancers, abnormal uterine bleeding, a history of stroke or venous thromboembolic disease, bone diseases or related conditions, use of hormones (estrogen, progestin, androgen) or corticosteroids within the previous six months and alcohol consumption of more than four drinks per day.

All participants received daily supplements of calcium (500 mg) and 400 to 600 IU of cholecalciferol (vitamin D-3). The women were randomly assigned to one of the following treatment protocols: raloxifene (60 mg/ twice daily), raloxifene (60 mg/once daily) and one placebo (once daily) and placebo (twice daily). Follow-up occurred every six months.

➤ **Cummings S, Duong T, Kenyon E, Cauley J, Whitehead M, and Krueger K (for the Multiple Outcomes of Raloxifene Evaluation (MORE) Trial.**

Serum estradiol level and risk of breast cancer during treatment with raloxifene. *Journal of the American Medical Association*, January 2002; 287:216–220. **Type:** Experimental (clinical trial)

Focus: An examination of the effect of raloxifene on the risk of breast cancer in women with high estradiol levels compared with women with low estradiol levels.

Conclusions: Raloxifene reduced the risk of breast cancer in postmenopausal women with high estradiol levels, but did not affect the risk of breast cancer in postmenopausal women with low estradiol levels.

Findings:

• Women in the placebo group with estradiol levels greater than 10 pmol/L had an increased risk of breast cancer: 6.80 times higher for women with high estradiol levels compared with women with low or undetectable estradiol levels.

• Women who had high estradiol levels (≥ 10 pmol/L) and received raloxifene had a 76 percent reduction in breast cancer risk.

• Raloxifene did not decrease the risk of breast cancer in women with low or undetectable estradiol levels.

• Raloxifene increased the risk of venous thromboembolisms and hot flashes in women despite their estradiol levels.

• Treatment with raloxifene reduced the risk of vertebral fractures.

Researchers' Comments: "If confirmed by other studies, measuring estradiol to determine breast cancer risk may help identify women likely to experience the greatest reduction in breast cancer risk form treatment with raloxifene" (220).

Participants and Methods: The MORE trial was placebo-controlled study designed to evaluate the hypothesis that raloxifene would reduce the risk of vertebral fractures in postmenopausal women with osteoporosis. This multicenter three-year study (1994–1998) conducted at 180 clinical centers in 25 countries was randomized and double-blind. A total of 7290 postmenopausal women aged 80 years or younger with osteoporosis formed the cohort of this study. The women were assessed for general health, medical conditions, mammography, reproductive history, bone density and estradiol levels. Women with a history of breast cancer were excluded. The participants were randomly assigned to receive raloxifene (60 mg/daily or 120 mg/daily) or placebo.

➤ **DiSaia P, Grosen E, Kurosaki T, Gildea M, Cowan B, and Anton-Culver H.**

Hormone replacement therapy in breast cancer survivors: a cohort study. *American Journal of Obstetrics and Gynecology*, May 1996; 174:1494–1498. **Type:** Observational (case-control)

Focus: An evaluation of the adverse effects of HRT on breast cancer survivors.

Conclusions: Hormone replacement therapy does not prevent adverse effects to breast cancer survivors. However, the researchers suggest the importance of conducting a randomized clinical trial to gather more information to study the issue. Moreover, they conclude that long-term studies will be needed to evaluate the effects of HRT plus tamoxifen on heart disease and osteoporosis.

Findings:
- The four-year disease-free rate was 74 percent in the HRT group and 86 percent in the control group.
- Analysis of survival time revealed no significance between the HRT and the control group.
- Disease-free time was not different between the two groups.

Researchers' Comments: "The benefits of hormone replacement therapy in preventing some degenerating processes in postmenopausal women cannot be denied. Patients must be informed so that they can make their own decisions regarding this important tool." (1497)

Participants and Methods: Forty-one women who had been diagnosed with breast cancer and who later received HRT were identified through hospital records. These women were matched with two controls (breast cancer patients) who had not received HRT using the population-based registry of the Cancer Surveillance Program of Orange County in California. Female breast cancer patients were selected for the control group on the basis of the following factors: age at diagnosis, stages of disease and year of diagnosis (1984–1992). The participants (HRT group) were assessed for history of cancer before the diagnosis of breast cancer. The type and duration of HRT were also evaluated. Follow-up information regarding recurrent disease and multiple primary cancer were obtained through physicians records. In the eighty-two control subjects, information on their history of cancer before diagnosis of breast cancer was determined through the population-based cancer registry. Information of the development of subsequent disease was determined through the cancer registry and by physician contact. Most of the HRT group received 0.625 mg/daily of conjugated estrogen or its equivalent plus *medroxyprogesterone* 2.5 mg/daily.

➤ **Ewertz M.**

Influence of non-contraceptive exogenous and endogenous sex hormones on breast cancer in Denmark. **The International Journal of Cancer**, December 1988; 42:832–838. **Type:** Observational (case-control)

Focus: An evaluation of the influence of sex hormones on the risk of breast cancer.

Conclusions: Sex hormones increase a woman's risk of breast cancer. A late *menarche* protects against breast cancer in premenopausal women. Continued menstrual cycles after the age of 50 increases a woman's risk of breast cancer. HRT also increases ones risk of breast cancer, and certain combinations of sex hormones may exert a greater influence on the risk than unopposed estrogen. The risk of breast cancer increases the longer the duration of HRT.

Findings:
• Pre-menopausal women had a decreased breast cancer risk with a later age at *menarche.*
• Natural menopause at an older age increases a woman's risk of breast cancer.
• The risk of breast cancer was higher with increasing duration of HRT use in all women studied except those women with an induced menopause.
• An approximately 30 percent increased breast cancer risk was observed in post-menopausal women who had used HRT.
• Women who had been treated with combined therapy (estrogen + *progestogen)* had an increased risk of breast cancer (**relative risk estimate:** 1.41 for combined sequential HRT/ 1.33 for combined therapy of other regimens).

Researchers' Comments: "The lack of an association found between breast cancer and body mass may be due to a misclassification bias" (837).

Participants and Methods: The researchers gathered information on 1486 cases of breast cancer diagnosed over a one year period. The information was obtained from the files of the national clinical trial of the

Danish Breast Cancer Cooperative Group and the Danish Cancer Registry. The cases consisted of 1,694 women (less than 70 years) diagnosed with breast cancer in Denmark between March 1983 and February 1984. The control group, women of various ages, was selected randomly and consisted of 1336 women from the general population. Questionnaires were used to assess various risk factors and the use of estrogen..

➤ Gapstur S, Morrow M, and Sellers T.

Hormone replacement therapy and risk breast cancer with a favorable histology: results of the Iowa Women's Health Study. *Journal of the American Medical Association*, June 1999; 281:2091–2097. **Type:** Observational (cohort)

Focus: An investigation of the association between HRT, breast cancer incidence and type of breast cancer.

Conclusions: Use of HRT was associated with an increased risk of invasive breast cancer.

Findings:
- A positive association between age at first birth and breast cancer risk was observed for all tumor types.
- Duration of HRT use was associated with an increased risk of an invasive carcinoma; however, these tumors had a "favorable histology" (*relative risk:* 1.44 for past users for five years or less/ 4.42 for current users for five years or less/1.00 for nonusers).
- Invasive or lobular breast cancer was slightly associated with current users of HRT (*relative risk:* 1.38 for five years or lesss/1.16 for five years or less/1.00 for nonusers).
- *Ductal* or *lobular carcinoma* were associated with an increased body mass index. Based on all tumor types, women who have used HRT for five or more years had in increased risk of breast cancer (*relative risk:* 1.11 for users/1.00 for nonusers).
- Based on all tumor types, women who had used HRT for five years or less had a slight increased risk of breast cancer (*relative risk:* 1.07 for users/1.00 for nonusers).

Researchers' Comments: "In this study, we could not determine the effect of type of HRT because data regarding the type of postmenopausal hormones used (ie, combined estrogen-progesterone vs. estrogen alone) were not available from the 1986 baseline questionnaire" (2097).

Participants and Methods: The participants were postmenopausal women aged 55 to 69 years who were part of the Iowa Women's Health Study, an eleven-year prospective study conducted from 1986 to

1996 involving 37,105 women. Breast cancer cases (1502 women) were identified using the Health Registry of Iowa. The participants were selected randomly from the 1985 Iowa Department of Transportation Drivers's license list. Women were excluded if they were premenopausal, had a history of breast cancer or mastectomy. The women were assessed at baseline for socioeconomic factors, cigarette and alcohol consumption, diet, general health, medical conditions, family medical history, reproductive history and estrogen use (duration). Four follow-up questionnaires were mailed in 1987, 1989, 1992 and 1997 to collect and update information. With the second follow-up survey the participants were asked if they had undergone mammography and length of time since last mammography. Breast cancer tumors were typed according to their histology and prognosis. Women who had used HRT were more likely to have had a mammogram within one year before the survey.

➤ Gambrell R, Maier R, and Sanders B.

Decreased incidence of breast cancer in postmenopausal estrogen-progestogen users. *Obstetrics and Gynecology*, Oct.–Dec. 1983; 62: 435–443. **Type:** Observational (cohort)

Focus: An examination of the incidence of breast cancer and endometrial cancer in women who used combined estrogen-progestogen therapy after menopause.

Conclusions: Estrogen replacement therapy does not increase the risk of breast cancer and possibly offers some protection. The addition of progestogen to estrogen therapy reduces the risk of breast cancer.

Findings:

- Estrogen plus progestogen (combined therapy) offers protection against breast cancer and endometrial cancer.
- Women who used combined therapy (estrogen + progestin) had a lower relative risk of breast cancer than nonusers (**relative risk:** 0.30 for users/1.00 for nonusers).
- Adding progestogen to postmenopausal estrogen therapy decreases the risk of breast cancer.

Researchers' Comments: "Because breast cells are not cyclicly shed by progestogens, the probable protective mechanism of progestogens is most likely at the intracellular level through changes in receptors and enzymatic activity" (441).

Subjects and Methods: The study took place in San Antonio, Texas at the Wilford Hall USAF Medical Center from 1975 to 1981. The female subjects were military personnel and military wives. For seven years

5,563 postmenopausal women were followed. The average age of the women in the study was 56.8 years. These women were monitored and assessed for health and socioeconomic status. The subjects with breast and endometrial cancer were identified from a tumor registry. During the study 53 participants developed cancer.

➤ Hiatt R, Bawol R, Fiedman G, and Hoover R.

Exogenous estrogens and breast cancer after bilateral oophorectomy, *Cancer*, July 1984; 54:139–144. **Type:** Observational (case-control)

Focus: An examination of the relationship between the development of breast cancer in women who had their ovaries surgically removed and the use of HRT.

Conclusions: Breast cancer risk was not increased in women who had undergone an oophorectomy and subsequently used HRT. The risk of breast cancer was lower than the risk of endometrial cancer. Women who had used conjugated estrogens had a higher risk of breast cancer.

Findings:
• Women with the most chart notations of estrogen or who used conjugated estrogens had a higher risk of breast cancer.
• No increased risk of breast cancer was found in women who had a longer duration of HRT.
• No increased risk of breast cancer was associated with higher doses of estrogen.
• Compared with nonusers, women who used estrogen had an increased risk of breast cancer (*relative risk estimate:* 1.10 for users of conjugated estrogens/2.50 for users of diethylstilbestrol.

Researchers' Comments: "Because of the small size of the group who never used estrogen, our study lacked statistical power for the comparison between that group and women who had ever used estrogen" (142).

Participants and Methods: The participants were recruited from a large prepaid health plan and follow-up resulted from use of medical records. Records of operations performed in all Northern California Kaiser Foundation Health Plan hospitals were the source of data for this study. The cases were 119 women (oophorectomized) who developed breast cancer and had used HRT. The cases were selected from hospital records of discharges (1960; 1971–1979). The control subjects were selected from the file of oophorectomized women in order to match each case. The cases and the controls were matched for age, date of oophorectomy, kind and dosage of estrogen. In all 3,537 women with breast cancer were identified.

➤ **Hoover R, Gray L, Cole P, and MacMahon B.**

Menopausal estrogens and breast cancer. Menopausal estrogens and breast cancer. *The New England Journal of Medicine*, August 1976; 295:401–405. **Type:** Observational (cohort)

Focus: An examination of the relationship between the use of conjugated estrogens during menopause and the development of breast cancer.

Conclusions: The use of estrogen during menopause does not protect against breast cancer. The relationship between estrogen use, *benign breast disease* and breast cancer may be cause for concern.

Findings:

• Women with a history of benign breast disease showed a higher relative risk of breast cancer compared to women without such a history; especially, those women who had developed the disease after they had started HRT.

• Women who had used HRT for more than 15 years had an increased risk of breast cancer compared to nonusers (**relative risk:** 2.00 for users/1.00 for nonusers).

• Women who used HRT had a 30 percent increased risk of breast cancer compared to women who never used HRT (**relative risk:** 1.30 for users/1.00 for nonusers).

• Women who had received HRT on an other than daily basis had an elevated risk of breast cancer.

• Two factors (*multiparity and oophorectomy*), normally are related to low risk of developing breast cancer, did not lower the risk for women who had taken estrogen for ten years or more.

• Women who had used higher-dose estrogen had an increased risk of breast cancer.

Researchers' Comments: "Although the data do not by themselves indict exogenous estrogens as a cause of breast cancer, they raise this risk as a definite possiblilty and indicate that a thorough evaluation is necessary" (405).

Participants and Methods: A total number of 1891 Caucasian women were recruited from a private practice in Kentucky to participate in the study. The average age at the start of HRT was 49 years and the average year at which observation was begun was 1958. The close of the study was in December 1972. Follow-up was conducted by questionnaires and phone calls to obtain relevant data. At the close of the study 1573 women were alive, 132 were dead and 186 were lost. The study time per women averaged 12 years and 620 women were followed for longer than 15 years. The control group consisted of women from the general population.

➤ Horwitz R and Stewart K.

Effects of clinical features on the association of estrogens and breast cancer, *The American Journal of Medicine*, February 1984; 76:192–198. **Type:** Observational (case-control)

Focus: An investigation of whether or not differences in HRT users could account for variability in breast cancer risk.

Conclusions: The use of HRT by postmenopausal women did not increase the risk of breast cancer. However, women who used HRT after an oophorectomy, did have an increased risk of breast cancer.

Findings:

• Breast cancer patients and control patients with benign breast disease who had undergone mammography and had used estrogen therapy, had a lower risk of breast cancer than "normal" control patients who had undergone mammography.

• Breast cancer patients and control patients who had undergone a biopsy and had used estrogen therapy had the lowest risk of breast cancer.

• Women who used HRT for hot flashes or after an oophorectomy, had an increased risk of breast cancer.

• Women using estrogen therapy for hot flashes or oophorectomy and who had undergone a biopsy had an increased risk of breast cancer (*odds ratio:* 1.50 for users/1.00 for nonusers).

• Women using HRT for vaginal atrophy, osteoporosis and aged skin did not have an increased risk of breast cancer.

Researchers' Comments: "The risk estimate varies according to the reason for the diagnostic breast procedure. We cannot establish whether the varying results reflect biologic differences in the patients subgroups or are a result of selection factors in the assembly of the case and control groups" (197).

Participants and Methods: Postmenopausal women, age 43 or older, were evaluated at Yale–New Haven Hospital from 1976 to 1979. Data from hospital and physician records were obtained regarding 257 breast cancer cases including their medical history and estrogen use. The researchers analyzed the results of each patient according to the reason for HRT (e.g., hot flashes, oophorectomy.) and the reason for mammography. To reduce the effect of selection bias, they selected breast cancer patients and separate control patients using breast mammography and breast biopsy. To compare these results with those of traditional sampling methods, the researchers assembled a control group of women hospitalized for medical or surgical conditions. Women who had a history of gynecologic malignancy (e.g., carcinomas of the ovary, breast, uterus or cervix) were excluded from the study.

> ➤ **Jick H, Walker A, Watkins R,**
> **D'Ewart D, Hunter J, Danford A,**
> **Madsen S, Dinan B, and Rothman K.**

Replacement estrogens and breast cancer. *American Journal of Epidemiology*, November 1980; 112:586–594. **Type:** Observational (case-control)

Focus: An evaluation of the relation between HRT and breast cancer in menopausal women.

Conclusions: HRT does not increase the risk of breast cancer in women who have had a hysterectomy and/or a oophorectomy. However, the risk of breast cancer is increased in women who have had a natural menopause and have used HRT.

Findings:

- An increase in the risk of breast cancer was found in women who had used HRT and had a natural menopause.
- Differences were found in the relative risk for breast cancer in estrogen users who had a natural menopause (**relative risk estimate:** 10.2 for 45–54 year old women/1.90 for 55–64 year old women).
- Current HRT users had an increased risk of breast cancer.
- Women who had hysterectomies (HRT users and nonuser) had a lower risk of breast cancer than women who had a natural menopause.
- Past use of HRT was not an important risk factor for developing breast cancer.

Researchers' Comments: "We believe it can safely be assumed that if there is any increased risk of breast cancer among hysterectomized women who use exogenous estrogens, it is modest.... The situation in natural menopause is less clear" (592).

Participants and Methods: The women in this study were selected from the Group Health Cooperative of Puget Sound, Washington. The researchers obtained the data from the Commission of Professional and Hospital Activities–Professional Activity Study (CPHA-PAS), a local tumor registry and computerized pharmacy records. The researchers identified 139 women (45–64 years) who were diagnosed with breast cancer from 1975 to 1978. Women were excluded from the study who had prior cancer or who were premenopausal. The cases were age matched to controls, 139 menopausal women (45–64 years) without breast cancer. The control group was also selected from women being hospitalized for acute illness or elective surgery during the same time as the women with breast cancer. All participants were assessed for general health, medical conditions, estrogen use, reproductive history. The women were stratified into two groups, hysterectomized and natural menopause.

➤ **Kaufman D, Miller D, Rosenberg L, Helmrich S, Stolley P, Schottenfeld D, and Shapiro S.**

Noncontraceptive estrogen use and the risk of breast cancer. *Journal of the American Medical Association*, July 1984; 252:63–77. **Type:** Observational (case-control)

Focus: An examination of the relationship between the risk of breast cancer and the use of noncontraceptive estrogens (HRT).

Conclusions: HRT does not increase the overall risk of breast cancer; however, some users may be at greater risk of breast cancer. Conjugated estrogen did not have an adverse effect in premenopausal or postmenopausal women, even among women who had undergone an oophorectomy.

Findings:

• Neither high nor low dose estrogen use was associated with an increased risk of breast cancer.
• *Nulliparous* women who had used HRT had an increased risk of breast cancer (**relative risk estimate:** 1.40 for users/1.00 for nonuser).
• Conjugated estrogens did not increase the risk of breast cancer in postmenopausal women.
• Women who had used HRT for a long time did not have an increased risk of breast cancer.
• No increase in the risk of breast cancer was found when women were grouped according family history, age at menopause, and age at first pregnancy.
• A 10 percent increased risk of breast cancer was found in women who had a history of cystic breast disease and used HRT (**relative risk estimate:** 1.10 for users/1.00 for nonusers).

Researchers' Comments: "The confidence intervals in some of the categories were wide enough to include the possibility of modest increases in risk" (67).

Participants and Methods: This study was based on hospital interviews conducted between July 1976 and June 1981 in various urban areas in the United States and Canada: Boston, New York, Philadelphia, Baltimore, Kansas City, Tucson, San Francisco and London, Ontario. The case and control groups were assessed for information on general health, medical history, medications and menopausal status. The cases were women less than 70 years with a primary diagnosis of breast cancer no more than six months before admission. The case group included 1,610 women with the median age of 51 years. The control group were women less than 70 years of age who were admitted to the hospital for nonmalignant conditions and had no history of cancer. Since many controls were young, one control was selected at random from the same decade of age as each case. The final control group was composed of 1,606 women with the median age of 51 years. The analysis was of women who had taken estrogen at least 18 months before admission to the hospital. Conjugated estrogen was taken by seventy percent of the HRT users. Other estrogens included diethylstilbestrol, estrone sulfate, ethinyl cream, unspecified estrogens and unspecified female hormones.

➤ **Kaufman D, Palmer J, Mouzon J, Rosenberg L, Stolley P, Warshauer M, Zauber A, and Shapiro S.**

Estrogen replacement therapy and the risk of breast cancer: results from case-control surveillance study. *The American Journal of Epidemiology*, May 1991; 134:1375–1385. **Type:** Observational (case-control)

Focus: An investigation of the relationship between HRT and the risk of breast cancer in postmenopausal women.

Conclusions: The use of unopposed conjugated estrogens did not increase the risk of breast cancer in most women who had used the therapy for short, moderate or long duration, but combined therapy did increase the risk.

Findings:
• No increased risk of breast cancer was found in current users of HRT (estrogen alone) after intervals as long as 15 years.
• No increase in the risk of breast cancer was found based on dose level.
• An increased risk of breast cancer was found for five or more years of HRT use in women with a low body mass index.
• Women who used combined therapy (estrogen + progestin) had a 70 percent increased risk of breast cancer compared to nonusers (*relative risk estimate:* 1.70 for users/1.00 for nonusers).

Researchers' Comments: "The possibility remains that the risk is modestly increased after very long duration of use, and that opposed therapy, and other noncontraceptive estrogens increase the risk" (1384).

Participants and Methods: Data was collected from the Case-Control Surveillance Study which was started in 1976. A comparison was made between 1989 cases and 2,077 hospital control subjects. In this group, 1,120 had non-gynecologic cancers and 957 had nonmalignant (non-gynecologic) conditions. Interviews took place in hospitals in the U.S. and Canada from 1980 to 1986. The cases were postmenopausal women 40–49 years old with breast cancer diagnosed not more than six months before their hospital admission and with no concurrent or previous cancer. Of the 1686, the median age was 59 years and 86 percent were Caucasians. The cases were age-matched with controls, 2,077 postmenopausal women (40–69 years) with malignant and nonmalignant conditions unrelated to estrogen use. There were 1,120 cancer controls including patients with colorectal cancer, malignant melanoma and various other cancers diagnosed within six months of admission and no other concurrent or previous cancer. There were 957 noncancer controls with no history of cancer.

➤ **LaVecchia C, Decarli A, Parazzini F, Gentile A, Liberati C, and Franceschi S.**

Non-contraceptive Oestrogens and the risk of breast cancer in women. *International Journal of Cancer*, December 1986; 38:853–858. **Type:** Observational (case-control)

Focus: An investigation of the relationship between the use of HRT and the risk of breast cancer

Conclusions: Breast cancer risk increased with HRT. The risk was more pronounced with longer use

Findings:

- The risk of breast cancer increased with longer duration of HRT.
- Women who used HRT for more than two years, had an increased risk of breast cancer (*relative risk estimate:* 2.04 for users/1.00 for nonusers).
- No important relationships were detected concerning parity, age at first birth, history of benign breast disease or family history of breast cancer.
- Women who had a natural menopause had a trend in terms of risk which increased with longer use of HRT.

Researchers' Comments: "The use of estrogen replacement therapy in Italy is considerably less frequent than in North American populations, where most other studies had been conducted" (856).

Participants and Methods: This study was initiated in 1983 in Milan, Northern Italy. Interviewers identified and questioned 1,108 women with breast cancer who were admitted for hospitalization. The cases included women (26–74 years old) with confirmed breast cancer, diagnosed within a year before the interview. The cases were matched with controls, women admitted for hospitalization for various conditions. The women had diseases which were not malignant, hormonal or gynecological. The controls included 1,281 women (25–74 years). These women were admitted for traumatic conditions: fractures, non-traumatic orthopedic disorders, acute surgical conditions and other illnesses (ear, nose, throat or dental disorders). The controls and cases were assessed for dietary habits, general health, reproductive history, mediations, medical conditions and estrogen use. The cases and controls were not age or geographically matched.

▶ Lawson D, Hershel J, Hunter J, and Madsen S.

Exogenous estrogens and breast cancer. *American Journal of Epidemiology*, November 1981; 114:710–713. **Type:** Observational (cohort)

Focus: An investigation of the interrelationship of age, HRT and breast cancer.

Conclusions: Current use of HRT increased the risk of breast cancer in middle-aged women who were premenopausal or naturally menopausal. From 1975 to 1979 a fall was observed in conjugated estrogen use in women age 45–54 years in the study cohort. There was also a drop in the overall incidence of breast cancer since 1977 in this group. During this time period, breast cancer rates in women who were not current users of HRT remained stable. This suggests that the fall in breast cancer rates documented in this study may be a result of decreased use of HRT by these women.

Findings:
- The rate of breast cancer for older (55–64 years) or younger (30–44 years) women was consistent from 1972 to 1979 with decreasing estrogen use.
- The rate of breast cancer for middle-aged women dropped with decreasing HRT use.

Researchers' Comments: "The present results provide additional evidence to support the hypotheses that current estrogen use increases the risk of breast cancer in middle-aged women who are premenopausal or naturally menopausal while having little, if any effect in younger and older women." (712).

Participants and Methods: A health maintenance organization, the Group Health Cooperative of Puget Sound, in Seattle, Washington was the source of participants in this study. Using computer files, the researchers identified women age 30–64 years with a diagnosis of breast cancer who were treated by mastectomy from 1972 to 1979. Women were excluded who had a history of previous breast cancer in the other breast or any other malignant condition. The researchers used the data to estimate the incidence rates of breast cancer for women from 1972 to 1979 in these age groups: 30–44 years, 45–54 years and 55–64 years. They also determined the incidence rates of breast cancer for women age 45–54 years who had used estrogen (including oral contraceptives and HRT), and nonusers of HRT for the years 1977–1979. Pharmacy files were used to determine the number of women using estrogen annually.

> ### Lipworth L, Katsouyanni K, Stuver S, Samoli E, and Hankinson S.

Oral contraceptives, menopausal estrogens, and the risk of breast cancer a case-control study in Greece, *The International Journal of Cancer*, September 1995; 62:548–551. **Type:** Observational (case-control)

Focus: An examination of the association between the use of oral contraceptives and menopausal estrogens and the risk of breast cancer.

Conclusions: An increased relative risk for breast cancer exists among menopausal estrogen users. This study did not find a significant trend of increasing risk of breast cancer with increasing duration of HRT.

Findings:
- Women who had used oral contraceptives did not have an elevated risk of breast cancer. This result was not dependent on duration of use and was not related to the time a woman had a first full term pregnancy.
- The longer, younger women had used oral contraceptives, the lower their risk of breast cancer.
- Women who had used HRT had an increased risk of breast cancer compared with nonusers (**odds ratio:** 1.52 for users/1.00 for nonusers).
- Long-term use of HRT increased a woman's risk of breast cancer (**odds ratio:** 1.42 for users/1.00 for nonusers).

Researchers' Comments: "The overall prevalence of oral contraceptives or menopausal estrogen use was low in this study, thereby limiting the statistical power of analysis among subgroups such as long term users. Moreover, due to small numbers, we were unable to evaluate the association between various aspects of use, including latency or recency of use and breast cancer risk" (550).

Participants and Methods: From January 1989 to December 1991, women recently diagnosed with breast cancer in four hospitals in Athens, Greece were identified as cases in the study. The cases included 820 patients. Two control groups were selected for each case. The total number of controls included 795 orthopedic patient controls and 753 healthy visitor controls. All the participants were assessed for general health, medical conditions, medications, estrogen use and reproductive status. In evaluating the role of menopausal estrogens, the analysis was limited to perimenopausal and postmenopausal women. Detailed information about the types of oral contraceptives or HRT used was not available.

➤ Mills P, Beeson W, Phillips R, and Frazer G.

Prospective study of exogenous hormone use and breast cancer in a Seventh-day Adventist. **Cancer**, August 1989; 64:591–597. **Type:** Observational (cohort)

Focus: An evaluation of the risk of breast cancer in women who reported use of both oral contraceptives and HRT.

Conclusions: The cumulative effect of both oral contraceptives and HRT may influence the development of breast cancer. The relative risk of breast cancer was elevated with increasing exposure to oral contraceptives and HRT. But no consistent trend was identified in this study in regard to high-risk and low-risk subgroups.

Findings:

- The highest risk for breast cancer was found in those women with less than one year of HRT use and those with six to ten years of use (***relative risk:*** 2.28 for one year or more/2.75 for 6–10 years/1.00 for nonusers).
- The highest risk associated with current use of hormone replacement therapy was in women who had a history of benign breast disease.
- Among women with a natural menopause there was no clear pattern between duration of HRT use and breast cancer risk.
- Naturally menopausal women who used HRT had a higher breast cancer risk than did women who received hysterectomies.
- Current users of HRT had a higher risk of breast cancer than non-users (***relative risk:*** 2.53 for current users/1.00 for nonusers).

Researchers' Comments: "Before 1976 estrogen doses were generally high (1.25 mg/day), taken for long periods of time and in a noncyclic fashion. The addition of progestin was not yet common. Therefore, the results of this study pertaining to HRT practices could show greater effect on breast cancer risk in comparison to current practices" (595).

Participants and Methods: This was a large cohort study involving Seventh-day Adventist women in which information was obtained from women by questionnaire in 1971. The women were assessed for general health, medial conditions, medications, HRT, oral contraceptive use and reproductive history. These women were followed for breast cancer and other diseases until the end of 1982. Follow-up surveillance consisted of annual mailings to subjects in the cohort obtaining information on hospitalization and other important factors. Tumor registries from computerized records from throughout the state were also accessed and used to detect cases in the geographic area of interest.

➤ **Newcomb P, Longnecker M, Storer B, Mittendorf R, Baron J, Clapp R, Bogdan G, and Willett W.**

Long-term hormone replacement therapy and the risk of breast cancer in postmenopausal women. *The American Journal of Epidemiology*, October 1995; 142:788–795. **Type:** Observational (case-control)

Focus: An investigation of the relationship between HRT and the risk of breast cancer.

Conclusions: The risk of breast cancer was similar in women who had used postmenopausal hormones and women who had never used any hormones. Neither duration of use nor kind of hormone was associated with an increased risk of breast cancer.

Findings:
• Users of estrogen or combined therapy (estrogen + progestin) had a relative risk of breast cancer similar to nonusers (**relative risk estimate:** 1.05 for users/1.00 for nonusers).
• No increased risk of breast cancer was found in those women who had used HRT for a long duration.
• Compared with controls, postmenopausal women with breast cancer were inclined to have a family history of breast cancer, report a history of benign breast disease, were mostly nulliparous, were older at the time of giving birth, consumed more than two alcoholic beverages a day, had greater body mass and were less likely to have had a surgical menopause.

Researchers' Comments: "Despite these null findings laboratory evidence consistently implicates estrogen as a promoter of mammary tumors" (794).

Participants and Methods: This study obtained data from 3,130 breast cancer cases and 3,698 controls interviewed between 1989 and 1991. Information on 6,888 women was available for analysis. The cases included females (less than 75 years) residing in Wisconsin, Western Massachusetts, Maine and New Hampshire with a diagnosis of invasive breast cancer. Cases were selected by each state's cancer registry for April 1989 through December 1991. The controls were randomly selected from a list of licensed drivers (less than 65 years) and from a roster of Medicare beneficiaries (65–74 years). The controls had no prior history of breast cancer.

▶ **Normura A, Kolonel L, Hirohata T, and Lee J.**

The association of replacement estrogens with breast cancer. *International Journal of Cancer*, January 1986; 37:49–53. **Type:** Observational (case-control)

Focus: An examination of the relationship between HRT and breast cancer in two population groups in Hawaii (Caucasian and Japanese).

Conclusions: Breast cancer risk was not increased in the HRT Caucasian cases compared with the Caucasian controls. There was no increase in breast cancer in HRT Japanese cases versus Japanese controls. However, when comparing Japanese HRT users with neighborhood controls and nonusers, there was an increase risk of breast cancer. The researchers also found that certain subgroups of women were at higher risk of breast cancer: early age at menarche, late age at first childbirth, late age at menopause, family history of breast cancer and past history of benign breast disease were risk factors.

Findings:
- The risk of breast cancer for Caucasian women who used HRT was slightly greater than those Japanese women who used HRT for less than eight years (*risk ratio estimate:* 1.30 for Caucasian users/1.00 for Japanese users/1.00 for nonusers.
- Breast cancer risk did not increase with long-term HRT in either ethnic group, but Japanese long-term users had a higher risk of breast cancer compared with neighborhood controls (*risk ratio estimate:* 2.60 for Japanese users).
- An increased risk of breast cancer was associated with the following factors: family history of breast cancer, benign breast disease, early menarche, older age at first birth, a late menopause, nulliparity.

Researchers' Comments: "In the present study, a higher percentage of Caucasian than Japanese cases had taken replacement estrogens (59.0 percent vs. 53.6 percent), but the case-control findings clearly showed that differential estrogen use between the two ethnic groups could not account for any of their substantial difference in breast cancer risk" (51).

Participants and Methods: Japanese and Caucasian women (45 to 74 years) living in Hawaii formed the study group. The cases were initially diagnosed for breast cancer between 1975 and 1980 at one of seven community hospitals on the island of Oahu. The cases were identified through hospital records. The Hawaii Tumor Registry was also used to identify cases missed. The diagnosis of breast cancer in the cases was confirmed by histologic slides reviewed by pathologists. Each case was matched with one hospital and one neighborhood control who had no previous or current history of breast cancer. Cases and controls were matched according to the following factors: sex, ethnic origin, age within five years, Oahu residency. Hospital controls were also matched with cases on the basis of time of hospitalization and admitting hospital. The controls were hospitalized for a variety of diseases. Women who were admitted to the hospital for any cancer diagnosis or with benign breast disease were excluded from the study. Neighborhood controls were obtained from telephone directories and lived in the same census tract as the cases. The participants were assessed for general health, medical conditions, medications, HRT use (type and duration), reproductive history and benign breast disease history.

➤ **Palmer J, Rosenberg L, Clarke E, Miller D, and Shapiro S.**

Breast cancer risk after estrogen replacement therapy: results from the Toronto Breast Cancer Study. *The American Journal of Epidemiology*, December 1991; 134:1386–1395. **Type:** Observational (case-control)

Focus: An investigation of the relation between estrogen use and breast cancer.

Conclusions: No increased risk of breast cancer was associated with the short-term use of conjugated estrogen. However, the researchers noted the possibility of an increase in the risk of breast cancer associated with very long-term use.

Findings:

- The relative risk of breast cancer in users of conjugated estrogens was lower than nonusers except for long-term use (*relative risk estimate:* 1.40 for users of HRT for 15 or more years/1.00 for nonusers).
- Relative risks for most durations of use were close to 1.00.
- The estimated relative risk for the longest duration (more than 15 years) was elevated.
- The results of this study suggest that estrogen use of less than 15 years does not increase a woman's risk of breast cancer.
- Estrogens only users had an increased risk of breast cancer (*relative risk estimate:* 2.60 for users for five or more years/1.00 for nonusers).

Researchers' Comments: "Estrogens taken with progestogens are thought to present less of a risk of endometrial cancer than unopposed estrogens and the combination is increasingly being prescribed to postmenopausal women. It is not known what the effect will be on breast cancer risk both protective and adverse effects have been hypothesized" (1394).

Participants and Methods: This Canadian study conducted from 1982 to 1986 evaluated the relation of alcohol consumption to breast cancer; however, the study was structured in such a way that other factors, such as estrogen use were also studied. Because the researchers assessed a number of factors, participation was not limited to postmenopausal women. The study population included women less than 70 years of age who lived in Toronto. The cases consisted of 607 women less than 70 years of age who had diagnosed primary breast cancer no more than six months prior to interviews. The controls, 1,214 women, were selected from tax assessment rolls, and were interviewed to obtain information. The cases and controls were matched by neighborhood and decade of age. All the participants were assessed for demographic factors, general health, medical conditions, family history of breast cancer, reproductive history and HRT. Most of the participants in this study took conjugated estrogen; only 7 percent had taken estrogen plus progestin so the results are more applicable to users of unopposed estrogen.

➤ **Ross R, Paganini-Hill A, Gerkins V, Mack T, Pfeffer R, Arthur M, and Henderson B.**

A case-control study of menopausal estrogen therapy and breast cancer. *Journal of the American Medical Association*, April 1980; 243:1635–1639. **Type:** Observational (case-control)

Focus: An investigation of the relationship between estrogen therapy and breast cancer.

Conclusions: An increased risk of breast cancer was found in women who received high doses of conjugated estrogen for long-term HRT.

Findings:
- Long-term use of HRT (7 or more years) was associated with an increased risk of breast cancer.
- Women who had accumulated high dosages of conjugated estrogens had a higher risk of breast cancer than nonusers.
- Women who had benign breast disease and used estrogen were at a higher risk of breast cancer than women who used estrogen but did not have benign breast disease **(relative risk estimate: 5.70 for**

long-term users with benign breast/2.10 for long-term users without benign breast disease/1.00 for nonusers).
• Women who did not have ovaries and received HRT did not have an increased risk of breast cancer.

Researchers' Comments: "A woman undergoing natural menopause at age 50 years who receives 1.25 mg of replacement estrogen therapy daily for approximately three years would increase her lifetime probability of getting breast cancer by age 75 from 6 percent to 12 percent if no latency is required, to almost 10 percent if a five-year latency is required and to 9 percent allowing for a ten-year latency period, assuming risk after exposure to be otherwise unaffected. These are sizable increases and carry with them sizable differences in *mortality*" (1639).

Participants and Methods: The study population involved two retirement communities in the Los Angeles area. The subjects were all Caucasian. The cases were selected by searching the disease indices of local hospitals. The cases, 147 postmenopausal breast cancer patients (50 to 74 years) diagnosed between 1971 and 1977, had no previous history of breast cancer. The cases were matched with controls selected from a community roster, according to residency, ethnicity, birth date, marital status, menopausal status and other socioeconomic factors. All participants were assessed for general health, medical conditions, medications, reproductive history and estrogen use. Because there were differences in prescribing practices (dosage and type of HRT), the researchers calculated for each subject a single comprehensive measure of total conjugated estrogen exposure, total milligrams accumulated dose (TMD).

▶ **Schairer C, Lubin J, Troisi R, Sturgeon S, Brinton L, and Hoover R.**

Menopausal estrogen and estrogen-progestin replacement therapy and breast cancer risk. *Journal of the American Medical Association,* January 2000; 283:485–491. **Type:** Observational (cohort)

Focus: An investigation of the difference in the risk of breast cancer in women who used estrogen alone or combined therapy (estrogen + progestin).

Conclusions: Women who use combined therapy (estrogen + progestin) have a greater risk of breast cancer than women who use estrogen alone.

Findings:
• Women who received HRT(combined therapy) had a higher risk of breast cancer than women who received estrogen alone or nonusers

(*relative risk:* 1.20 for estrogen alone/1.40 for combined therapy/ 1.00 for nonusers).

- Lean women who received combined therapy (estrogen + progestin) were at greater risk of breast cancer than heavier women who received combined therapy. The *relative risk* among lean women increased by 0.12 percent for each year of use.
- Based on four years of use, an increased risk of breast cancer was observed in women who received HRT, estrogen alone or combined therapy (*relative risk:* 1.20 for estrogen alone/1.40 for combined therapy).
- Combined therapy (estrogen + progestin) was associated with a significant increase in the risk of invasive breast cancer.
- Women who received estrogen alone had an increased risk of breast cancer of 0.01 percent with each year of use; women who received combined therapy (estrogen + progestin) had an increased risk of breast cancer of 0.08 percent with each year of use.

Researchers' Comments: "We also found significant increased in risk for the vast majority of invasive tumors classified as lobular and/or ductal carcinomas, results that are not consistent with those of Gapstur et al. Their categories for duration of use (less or more than 5 years) may have obscured an effect of long-term use; in addition, they did not present results among lean women" (491).

Participants and Methods: Participants in this study were 46,355 postmenopausal women (86 percent Caucasian) enrolled in the Breast Cancer Detection Demonstration Project (BCDDP) conducted between 1973 and 1980 at twenty-nine screening centers throughout the United States were. This report presents follow-up data on this study, gathered from 1980 to 1995. The study involved the following groups: all screened participants who had breast surgery during the screening period but with no evidence of malignant disease; women who had been recommended for possible surgery but did not have either a biopsy or aspiration; a group of women who did not have surgery nor were recommended for possible surgery. The follow-up study was divided into three phases. The first two phases of the follow-up period were conducted through telephone interviews between 1979 and 1986, and one mailed questionnaire was employed between 1987 and 1989. The third phase of the follow-up, one mailed questionnaire, was used between 1993 and 1995. The purpose of follow-up research was to assess breast cancer risk factors, breast cancer screening practices (e.g., mammogram history), surgical procedures performed, and HRT use (type, dosage, duration). During the initial entry into the study, the participants were assessed for education and health data. Height and weight information was gathered at baseline and each screening visit. During follow-up, 2082 breast cancer cases were identified in the study population through self-reports or reports of breast cancer on death certificates. Conjugated estrogens (Premarin) and progestin (medroxyprogesterone acetate) were the HRT used most by the participants.

> ## Sherman B, Wallace R, and Bean J.

Estrogen use and breast cancer: interaction with body mass. **Cancer**, April 1983; 51:1527–1531. **Type:** Observational (case-control)

Focus: An examination of the relationship between estrogen use, body mass and breast cancer.

Conclusions: The risk of breast cancer is influenced by woman's weight. Women of low weight who had used HRT did not have an increased risk of breast cancer, but women who were overweight and had used HRT had an increased risk of breast cancer. However, the thin breast cancer patients who had used HRT were diagnosed with and appeared to develop breast cancer earlier than nonusers.

Findings:
- Thin women who used HRT had a lower risk of breast cancer than heavier women who used HRT (**relative risk estimate:** 0.36 for thin women/1.10 for heavier women).
- Thin women who used HRT developed breast cancer earlier and were diagnosed sooner than women who were of similar weight but had never used HRT.
- No significant relationship existed between body weight and age of the development of breast cancer in those women who never used HRT.
- Over weight women who used HRT did not development breast cancer any earlier than over weight women who did not use HRT.
- Breast cancer diagnosis averaged five years earlier in thin users than nonusers.

Researchers' Comments: "Obesity is associated with greater estrogen production from ... *precursors*, such as *androstenedione*. This may result in higher serum levels of estrogen, predominantly estrone. It is therefore possible that the interaction of weight and estrogen use is related to a more intense *estrogenic* environment in obese estrogen users" (1530).

Participants and Methods: This case control study, conducted between 1974 and 1978 at the University of Iowa Hospital, involved 113 postmenopausal breast cancer patients. The women were assessed for general health, medical conditions, reproductive history and estrogen use. Duration of estrogen use was determined, but dosages or specific HRT were not identified. Each case was aged-matched with a control patient selected from the medical and surgery wards of the hospital.

> ## Stanford J, Weiss N, Voigt L, Daling J, Habel L, and Rossing M.

Combined estrogen and progestin hormone replacement therapy in relation to risk of breast cancer in middle age women. *The Journal of the American Medical Association*, July 1995; 274:137–142. **Type:** Observational (case-control)

Focus: An investigation of the risk of breast cancer in relation to the use of combined therapy (estrogen + progestin).

Conclusions: Most women who received HRT did not have an increased risk of breast cancer regardless of the therapy used. No association was found between breast cancer and duration of HRT. However, the researchers found an elevated risk of breast cancer in women who had undergone a hysterectomy with both ovaries removed and who had used HRT (estrogen + progestin).

Findings:

• Negligible difference in risks were observed in various categories of family history of breast cancer, previous biopsies of benign breast disease, alcohol consumption and use of oral contraceptives.

• Women who used combined therapy did not have an increased risk of breast cancer (*relative odds:* 0.90 for users/1.00 for nonusers).

• A modest increased risks of breast cancer was found in thin women who used HRT, estrogen alone or combined therapy.

• Women who had undergone a hysterectomy, had both ovaries removed and used HRT (combined therapy) subsequently, showed an elevated risk of breast cancer.

• No increased risk of breast cancer was found for women who had used HRT for a long duration (more than 20 years).

Researchers' Comments: "If breast cancer incidence is affected by the use of estrogen-progestin HRT, and is such an effect requires 10 to 20 years to become manifest, our study could not identify such an effect" (141).

Participants and Methods: Cases (537) were identified through the Cancer Surveillance System, a population-based cancer registry that covers the 13 counties of Northwestern Washington state. They were Caucasian women (50–64 years old) who were diagnosed with histologically confirmed breast cancer between January 1988 and June 1990. The controls were 492 women, randomly selected from King County Washington with no history of breast cancer. The participants were assessed for general health, medical conditions, HRT, reproductive history and risk factors.

➤ **Steinberg K, Thacker S, Smith J, Stroup D, Zak M, Flanders W, and Berkelman R.**

A meta-analysis of the effect of estrogen replacement therapy on the risk of breast cancer. *Journal of the American Medical Association*, April 1991; 265:1985–1990. **Type:** Statistical (meta-analysis)

Focus: An investigation of the impact of the duration of estrogen replacement therapy on breast cancer risk.

Conclusions: Women who received HRT had an increased risk of breast cancer after five years of use. Long-term use increased the risk of breast cancer by about 30 percent. HRT increased the risk of breast cancer regardless of family history of breast cancer, parity, or history of benign breast disease.

Findings:
- Women who used HRT and had a family history of breast cancer had a higher risk of breast cancer.
- After 15 years of use, women who received HRT (mostly estradiol alone or combined therapy) had a 30 percent increased risk of breast cancer.
- Studies that included women with all types of menopause showed an increased risk of breast cancer for long-term use of HRT *(relative risk:* 1.30 for users/1.00 for never users).
- Estrogen use increased the risk of breast cancer in women who had oophorectomies.
- Breast cancer risk increased in studies that included premenopausal women *(relative risk:* 2.20 for users/1.00 for never users).

Researchers' Comments: "When we analyzed each group separately, high-scoring studies showed a significantly increased risk of breast cancer with increasing duration of estrogen use" (1987).

Participants and Methods: The researchers used MEDLINE CANCER LIT Current Contents, and EXCERPTA MEDIA databases for 1966 through September 1989 to find studies in which the effect of HRT on breast cancer was investigated. The researchers excluded studies that did not distinguish between noncontraceptive and contraceptive estrogens. Studies that included subjects with a previous history of breast cancer were also excluded. Studies which included postmenopausal women were analyzed separately. Each study was reviewed by three epidemiologist to assess the methods employed. The epidemiologist rated the studies on a scale of 0 to 100.

RATINGS OF VARIOUS STUDIES
(CASE-CONTROL AND COHORT)
BASED ON A 0 TO 100 POINTS*

Studies That Showed an Increased Risk of Breast Cancer	*Quality Score: High 71–83 Moderate 40–57 Low 15–38*
Jick et al., 1980	38 (low)
Ross et al., 1980	75 (high)
Hoover et al., 1981	72 (high)
Hulka et al., 1982	38 (low)
Hiatt et al., 1984	71 (high)
Nomura et al., 1986	57 (moderate)
Brinton et al., 1986	51 (moderate)
LaVecchia et al., 1986	43 (moderate)
Wingo et al., 1987	83 (high)
Bergkvist et al., 1989	82 (high)
Hoover et al., 1976	48 (moderate)

Studies That Showed No Increased Risk of Breast Cancer	*Quality Score*
Casagrande et al., 1976	12 (very low)
Sartwell et al., 1977	13 (very low)
Wynder et al., 1978	25 (low)
Ravinhar et al., 1979	26 (low)
Kelsey et al., 1981	40 (moderate)
Sherman et al., 1983	22 (low)
Horwitz and Stuart, 1984	23 (low)
Kaufman et al., 1984	45 (moderate)
McDonald et al., 1986	62 (moderately high)
Nachtigall et al., 1979	72 (high)
Bland et al., 1980	13 (very low)
Gambrell et al., 1983	33 (low)
Buring et al., 1987	57 (moderate)
DuPont et al., 1989	50 (moderate)

*(data from Steinberg et al, **JAMA**; April 1991; 265:1986–1988)

➤ Wingo P, Layde P, Lee N, Rubin G, and Ory H.

The risk of breast cancer in postmenopausal women who have used estrogen replacement therapy. *The Journal of the American Medical Association*, January 1987; 257:209–215. **Type:** Observational (case-control)

Focus: An examination of the relationship between HRT and breast cancer according to type of menopause.

Conclusions: HRT users had a slightly increased risk of breast cancer. Women without ovaries who had used HRT had a consistently elevated risk.

Findings:
- Women who had used HRT had a risk of breast cancer slightly higher than those women who had never used hormones.
- Women who had surgical menopause and removal of the ovaries had a slightly elevated risk of breast cancer.
- No dose-response relationship was found with breast cancer risk and HRT use.
- Compared with the control group, postmenopausal women with breast cancer were more often older at the time of their first full-term pregnancy or were nulliparous, had an early menarche, had a history of benign breast disease, and reported a first-degree relative who had breast cancer.
- Women who had used HRT for 15–19 years had a 30 percent greater risk of breast cancer than nonusers (***relative risk estimate:*** 1.30 for users/1.00 for nonusers).

Researchers' Comments: "Whether ovaries are removed or intact, the risk of breast cancer does not appear to increase with either duration or estrogen replacement of higher doses ... postmenopausal women and their physicians must balance the potential risks and benefits of ERT" (215).

Participants and Methods: The data collected for this study were obtained during the Cancer and Steroid Hormone Study. This study investigated the association between oral contraceptives, breast, ovarian and endometrial cancer. Analysis included 1369 cases and 1645 controls. The cases were women (20–54 years) living in eight geographic study locations. Tumor registries were used to identify women with newly diagnosed breast cancer between December 1980 and December 1982. The controls were women (20–54 years) from the same geographic area as the cases and selected randomly by digit dialing of residential telephone numbers. The women were interviewed in their homes for risk factors, HRT use and other health issues. Only the use of oral conjugated estrogen was evaluated because at the time of this study this was the major form of treatment.

2

Cardiovascular Conditions

Cardiovascular conditions include heart attack, stroke, hypertension, hyperlipidemia, diabetes, diseases of the blood vessels and insufficient delivery of blood to the organs. The term heart disease describes disease affecting the blood vessels and the heart. Heart disease causes 60 percent of the sudden deaths in women. Cardiovascular disease is the number one cause of death in the United States: coronary heart disease is number one cause of mortality and is the second leading cause of death in individuals between 45 and 64 years, and it is the number one cause of death in individuals over 65 years. Stroke is the third leading cause of death. Since 1984 the number of deaths in females due to cardiovascular conditions has exceeded those for male.

(http://www.american.heart.org)

Heart Disease Is Influenced by Many Variables

Heart disease involves a complex interplay of many factors: diet, physical activity, cigarette consumption, emotional response, genetics, blood pressure, cholesterol levels, triglycerides, C-reactive protein levels, homocysteine levels, viral and bacterial infections. Data from the ongoing Nurses' Health Study found that intake of foods containing hydrogenated transfats were significantly associated with a higher risk of coronary heart disease in women (Willett et al., 1993). This study also found that increasing physical exercise was strongly associated with a reduced risk of stroke (Hu et al., 2000), and smoking was the greatest risk factor for heart disease

55

(Stampfer et al., 2000). Other researchers have found an emotional connection to the development of heart disease: emotional stress, hostility and anger increase the risk of developing heart disease by raising blood pressure, cholesterol levels and coronary artery calcification (Iribarren et al., 2000). Depression and social isolation contribute to the development or progression of heart disease (Lavoie et al., 2000); whereas, Yoga, exercise and good coping skills can help a person lower the risk of heart disease (Ornish, 1993). Genetics plays a role in the development of heart disease. A group of researchers found that individuals with the MTHFR 677C →T genotype had a higher risk of cardiovascular conditions, especially if these individuals had low levels of folate in their blood (Klerk et al., 2002). Lowering total cholesterol and low-density lipoproteins (LDL) cholesterol reduces both fatal and nonfatal cardiac events (Ballantyne, 1998; Stark, 1996). C-reactive protein levels, viral and bacterial infections are other factors that can lead to arterial inflammation and possibly to heart disease (Schah et al., 2000).

HRT and Heart Disease

Does HRT prevent mortality from heart disease in older women? Earlier observational studies showed HRT lowered the risk of heart disease by lowering LDL cholesterol and raising HDL cholesterol. However, these studies used estrogen therapy (primarily Premarin) at dosages higher than current levels and provided data on estrogen alone therapy not combined therapy. The Women's Health Initiative clinical trial found that women who received combined therapy experienced an increase risk of heart attack and stroke even early in the study (Writing Group for the Women's Health Initiative Investigators, 2002). Even before the alarming results of the Women's Health Initiative, the American Heart Association (*Circulation*, July 2001) decided to recommend against prescribing HRT to prevent heart disease, citing conflicting studies and weak data supporting the heart protective benefits of HRT. The results form the HERS study (Hulley et al., 1998) surprised many researchers who thought that HRT might be used to treat heart disease: HRT (combined therapy) increased the risk of a coronary event in women with diagnosed heart disease. Estrogen therapy alone may affect women differently than combined therapy. The Women's Health Initiative is continuing the estrogen arm of its study, so results will be reported within the next few years.

Preventing Heart Disease:
Drug Treatments, Vitamin Therapies,
Controlling Blood Pressure, Diet and Exercise

Using statin drugs, niacin, aspirin, vitamin therapy and limiting consumption of dietary fats may lower the risk of heart disease or stroke by affecting LDL cholesterol, HDL cholesterol or clotting factors. Statin drugs (e.g., Zocor, Lipitor, Pravastatin) are effective at reducing the risk of coronary heart disease by lowering high LDL cholesterol. A meta-analysis of five clinical trials found a 31 percent reduction in major coronary events with statin drugs (LaRosa et al., 2000). Niacin, a B vitamin, has been shown to lower LDL cholesterol. The Cholesterol Lowering Atherosclerosis Study found that after four years of treatment with colestipol (a statin drug) plus niacin, participants had regression of coronary artery lesions. Aspirin protects the heart lowering the risk of strokes and fatal heart attacks by preventing clot formation (Chen et al., 2000; Garcia et al., 2000). Folic acid and vitamin E may protect the heart. Folic acid lowers homocysteine in the blood. Elevated levels of homocysteine have been associated with heart disease and stroke (Brattström et al., 1998; Schnyder et al., 2002). Vitamin E, an antioxidant, may protect the heart by preventing LDL cholesterol from oxidizing and depositing plaque in the arteries (Plotnick et al., 1997). However, not all studies have found that vitamin E is heart-protective (Fairfield et al., 2002). A study of postmenopausal women with coronary stenosis found no cardiovascular benefit from estrogen-progestin therapy, vitamin E or vitamin C therapy (Waters et al., 2002).

Having high blood pressure is a risk factor for heart disease. Treating blood pressure reduces the risk of hypertension-related death or disability. High blood pressure can be influenced by changing diet, getting regular exercise and managing stress. The Nurses' Health study found that age, weight and alcohol consumption were the strongest predictors of hypertension. Following a diet that is high in magnesium and fiber can lower blood pressure (Ascherio et al., 1996). Many hypertensive treatments exist, but the Antihypertensive and Lipid-Lowering Treatment to Prevent Heart Attack Trial (ALLHAT) found that diuretics were less expensive and superior to other forms blood-pressure treatments (ALLHAT Collaborative Research Group, 2002).

Regular exercise and a healthy diet can reduce the risk of heart disease (Page et al., 1996; Ornish, 1998). Consistent aerobic exercise increases HDL cholesterol, lowers blood pressure, reduces total cholesterol, burns calories and sustains cardiovascular fitness (Atalay & Sen, 1999). The Cholesterol Lowering Atherosclerosis Study found that increased consumption of all fats was associated with a significant risk of arterial lesions. One researcher has found that a very restrictive low fat diet (10 percent) fat can reverse the process of atherosclerosis (Ornish et al., 1998). A meta-analysis of 19 randomized clinical trials found that consuming less dietary fat led to a 5.7 percent reduction in cholesterol (Tang et al., 1998). Some studies suggest that changing the ratio of fat consumption, reducing saturated fats and eliminating hydrogenated fats while increasing polyunsaturated fats or monounsaturated fats can also reduce LDL cholesterol (Sarkinen et al., 1994). Some fats consumed moderately may benefit the cardiovascular system. Omega-3-fatty acid, a polyunsaturated fat found in flaxseed and fish, can raise HDL cholesterol and may prevent blood clot formation (Franceschini et al., 1991). Polyunsaturated and monounsaturated oils found in nuts and nut butter lower the risk of type two diabetes in women (Jiang et al., 2002; Willett & Stampfer, 2003). These fats may help regulate glucose and insulin levels in the blood: elevated levels of glucose or insulin increase the risk of type two diabetes and cardiovascular disease by raising triglycerides, lowering HDL cholesterol and increasing LDL cholesterol.

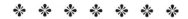

➤ **Baron Y, Galea R, and Brincat M.**

Carotid artery wall changes in estrogen-treated and -untreated postmenopausal women. ***Obstetrics and Gynecology***, June 1998; 91:982–985. **Type:** Experimental (clinical trial)

Focus: An examination of the effect of HRT on the thickness of the carotid artery.

Conclusions: HRT in postmenopausal women thickens the *carotid artery* and may therefore protect women from heart disease.

Findings:
• Women who had estradiol implants had the thickest carotid arteries (media and externa layers).
• Women who had received oral HRT had thicker media and externa layers in their carotid arteries than the control group (nonusers).
• Women who had received HRT had thinner intima layers than untreated women.

Researchers' Comments: "The direct effect of progesterone on vessel wall composition is not yet known" (985).

Participants and Methods: This small study involved 129 postmenopausal women recruited from the gynecology outpatient department at St. Luke's Hospital, Gwardamangia, Malta. The study was not randomized or blinded. Participants were assessed for general health, medical conditions, reproductive history, medications, HRT (type, dosage, duration). During recruitment women were excluded from the study if they had any condition that would affect their cardiovascular system, such as diabetes, high cholesterol, high blood pressure, high alcohol or cigarette consumption. The women were classified into three groups: forty-six women receiving oral HRT (conjugated estrogens, 0.625 mg/d + norgestrel, 1mg/d); thirty-two women receiving estradiol implants (100 mg) and women not receiving HRT. The mean duration of HRT use in both groups was 30 months. Measurements of the carotid artery were taken using an ultrasonic probe. Twenty measurements were taken in each women on four different occasions over two days. The ultrasonic method was also compared with histologic measurements of the carotid and iliac arteries of two cadavers to assure the validity of the ultrasonic method.

➤ **Barrett-Connor E, Grady D, Sashegyi A, Anderson P, Cox D, Hoszowski K, Rautaharju P, and Harper K (for the MORE Investigators).**

Raloxifene and cardiovascular events in osteoporotic postmenopausal women: four-year results from the MORE (Multiple Outcomes of Raloxifene Evaluation) randomized trial. *Journal of the American Medical Association*, February 2002; 287:847–857. **Type:** Experimental (clinical trial)

Focus: An investigation of the effect of raloxifene on cardiovascular events in postmenopausal women with osteoporosis.

Conclusions: Raloxifene therapy for four years did not significantly change the risk of cardiovascular events in most of the participants, except those women with an increased cardiovascular risk.

Findings:
- No significant difference in cardiovascular events was found in the overall cohort between the treatment group and the placebo group.
- Women who had an increased risk of cardiovascular events at baseline had a reduced risk of cardiovascular events with treatment with raloxifene (***relative risk:*** 0.60 for the raloxifene group—either 60 mg/d or 120 mg/d).
- Unlike estrogen therapy, no evidence suggested that raloxifene caused an early increase in the risk of cardiovascular problems.
- Raloxifene treatment reduced significantly levels of LDL, but not HDL cholesterol (5 percent reduction in total cholesterol).
- The number of cardiac events during the first year of treatment was

not significantly different in the overall cohort or among women at increased cardiovascular risk or with established heart disease.

Researchers' Comments: "Before raloxifene is used for prevention of CV events, these findings must be confirmed by an adequately powered, randomized trial with CV events as predefined outcomes" (857).

Participants and Methods: The MORE trial recruited 7705 postmenopausal women (31–81 years) with osteoporosis. The women were enrolled at 180 centers in twenty-five countries. Of the participants, 95.7 percent were Caucasian. The women were assessed for general health, medical history and medication use and blood chemistry. All the women received calcium and cholecalciferol supplements, which might have affected the risk of fractures in both placebo and raloxifene groups. Bone mineral density, using dual-energy X-ray absorptiometry at baseline and annually. Vertebral and fractures were assessed using radiography at baseline, 24 months and 36 months. Mammographies were performed at baseline, at one year (optional) and year two and three. The women were randomized into two study groups. Study group one included women who had hip and spine bone mineral density t-score below −2.5. The women in the second study group had low bone mineral density and had experienced one or more mild to severe vertebral fractures. Women were excluded for the following conditions: bone disease other than osteoporosis, severe postmenopausal symptoms or abnormal bleeding, endometrial, breast or skin cancer, a history of *thromboembolism*, estrogen use within the previous two months, androgen use or medication for osteoporosis within the past six months, abnormal liver tests or consumption of more than four alcoholic drinks per day. Within each study group, women were randomly assigned to receive a placebo, 60 mg/d raloxifene or 120 mg/d raloxifene. All the participants received 500 mg of calcium daily and 400 to 600-IU of cholecalciferol (vitamin D-3). The primary outcomes of the trial were bone mineral density and vertebral fractures. This study presents the data of a secondary analysis from the MORE trial. The main outcomes of this analysis were cardiovascular events including coronary event (myocardial infarction, unstable angina, or coronary ischemia) and cerebrovascular events (stroke or transient ischemic attack).

➤ **Bruschi F, Meschia M, Soma M, Perotti D, Paoletti R, and Crosignani P.**

Lipoprotein (a) and other lipids after oophorectomy and estrogen replacement therapy. **Obstetrics and Gynecology,** December 1996; 88: 950–954. **Type:** Experimental (clinical trial)

Focus: An assessment of the effect of surgical menopause and follow-up HRT on *lipoprotein (a)* and common lipids.

Conclusions: Surgical menopause affects the lipid profile. HRT can improve the lipid profile.

Findings:

- Oral conjugated estrogen improved lipid profile in women who had undergone an oophorectomy by lowering total cholesterol and *LDL cholesterol* and raising *HDL cholesterol.*
- Women who had an oophorectomy and received HRT had an increase in *triglyceride* levels.
- After a surgical menopause, lipoprotein (a) levels increased, total cholesterol increased, LDL cholesterol increased and HDL cholesterol decreased in the women.
- Women who had a surgical menopause did not have an increase in triglyceride levels.

Researchers' Comments: "The influence of the type and dosage of female sex hormones on the concentration of Lp(a) has not yet been determined" (953).

Participants and Methods: Twenty-four women, mean age of 48.3 years, were recruited at the Department of Obstetrics and Gynecology of the University of Milan, Italy from September 1993 to March 1994. The women were premenopausal, had not received HRT and had undergone a hysterectomy and bilateral oophorectomy for benign conditions. Before the surgery, the women were assessed for total cholesterol, low density lipoproteins (LDL cholesterol), high density lipoproteins (HDL cholesterol), triglycerides and *gonadotropins* (FSH, LH). These measurements were taken again one, two and three months postoperatively. In 19 women who volunteered for HRT, the lipid profile was assayed again at three, six and twelve months of treatment. Women who had alcoholism, cancer, liver, kidney or gastrointestinal diseases were excluded from the study.

➤ **Bush T, Barrett-Connor E,
Cowan L, Criqui M, Wallace R,
Suchindran C, Tyroler H, and Rifkind B.**

Cardiovascular mortality and noncontraceptive use of estrogen in women: results from the lipid research clinics program follow-up study. **Circulation**, June 1987; 75:1102–1109. **Type:** Observational (cohort)

Focus: An examination of the relationship between HRT and cardiovascular mortality.

Conclusions: Women who used HRT for the study period of 8.5

years had a lower risk of cardiovascular death than women not using estrogen. The heart protective effect of HRT may be in the raising of the good HDL cholesterol.

Findings:

- Nonusers of HRT had 44 deaths resulting from *cardiovascular disease*; users of HRT had 6 deaths related to cardiovascular disease.
- Women who received HRT had a lowered risk of cardiovascular disease (**relative risk:** 0.34 for users/1.00 for nonusers).
- The prevalence of cardiovascular disease was slightly higher in users of HRT than nonusers at *baseline.*
- Women who used HRT had a lower risk of death from all causes (**relative risk:** 0.54 for users/1.00 for nonusers).
- HRT use was associated with a lower risk of cardiovascular even after adjusting for age, blood pressure, and smoking.

Researchers' Comments: " A history of cigarette smoking was common among those who died from cardiovascular disease. Of the six estrogen users who died from cardiovascular disease, four were current smokers and two were former smokers...." (1105)

Participants and Methods: The participants were 2270 Caucasian women (40–69 years) who were followed for 8.5 years in the Lipid Research Clinics Programs Follow-up Study. The women in the study were part of the Lipid Research Clinics Prevalence Study of Cardiovascular Disease conducted in ten clinics in North American starting in 1972. The women were assessed for estrogen use, general health, medical conditions, medications, reproductive history, smoking, family history of cardiovascular disease, plasma lipids and blood pressure. Most of the women in this study had taken estrogen alone (conjugated equine estrogen—Premarin). Only six HRT users were taking combined therapy (estrogen + progestin). Women were excluded from the study if they reporting using oral contraceptives, had incomplete data regarding a hysterectomy and inconsistent information on questions pertaining to menstrual history.

➤ Christ M, Seyffart K, and Wehling M.

Attenuation of heart-rate variability in postmenopausal women on progestin-containing hormone replacement therapy (Research Letters). *The Lancet*, June 1999; 353:1939–1940. **Type:** Observational (case-control)

Focus: An investigation of the effect of HRT on *heart-rate variability* in postmenopausal women.

Conclusions: HRT (combined therapy) lowers heart rate variability in healthy postmenopausal women. A reduced HRV is associated with an increased risk of cardiovascular mortality.

Findings:
- Mean blood pressure was not affected by HRT.
- Heart rate was increased in women who received combined therapy (estrogen + progestin).
- Women who received combined therapy (estrogen + progestin) had a significantly lower HRV than controls or women who received HRT (estrogen alone).
- Women who did not receive HRT and women who received HRT (estrogen alone) had similar HRV measurements.

Researchers' Comments: "Hormone replacement therapy may attenuate heart rate variability in healthy postmenopausal women, and a reduced HRV could indicate an increased risk of cardiovascular mortality. This, effect, however appears to be restricted to HRT containing progestins. Thus, the addition of progestins in HRT may outweigh postulated beneficial effects of *oestrogens* on cardiovascular risks. These observations could explain at least in part the disappointing results of combined oestrogen/progestin HRT in secondary prevention of coronary artery disease reported recently (HERS Study)" (1940).

Participants and Methods: This German study involved 45 healthy postmenopausal women (48–71 years) who had used or not used HRT for at least three months. The study group was randomly selected from 193 volunteers. The women were assessed form general health, medications, medical conditions, reproductive history, and estrogen use. Women receiving drug therapy or having diseases that affect the *autonomic system* (e.g., diabetes) were excluded. Measures of HRV (heart rate, TP, SDNN) and measures of vagal tone (pNN50, RMSSD) were recorded.

> ➤ **Daly E, Vessey M, Hawkins M,**
> **Carson J, Gough J, and Marsh S.**

Risk of venous thromboembolism in users of hormone replacement therapy. **The Lancet**, October 1996; 348:977–980. **Type:** Observational (case-control)

Focus: An investigation of whether current use of HRT is associated with venous thromboembolism.

Conclusions: Current HRT use is associated with a increased risk of venous thromboembolism.

Findings:
- Current use of HRT is associated with an increased risk of *venous*

thromboembolism (**odds ratio:** 3.60 for current users/1.00 for non-users).

- No increased risk of venous thromboembolism was found in past users of HRT
- The highest risk of venous thromboembolism was found in short-term current HRT users.
- Current users of HRT had a risk which was three times greater than nonusers.

Researchers' Comments: "The annual rate of *idiopathic* VTE per 100,000 women ages 45–64 is estimated to be 27.4 among HRT users and 10.9 among non-users, which gives an annual total of 16.5 cases per 100,000 that may be attributed to using HRT. This risk may be entirely acceptable to women using HRT in the short-term for relief of menopausal symptoms, especially to those without other risk factors for VTE. For long-term HRT users, these findings need to be weighed against the probable benefits of long-term treatment" (980).

Participants and Methods: During this study 108 cases and 232 controls were recruited from February 1993 to December 1994 from hospitals in Oxford, England. Eligible cases were women (45–64 years) with a suspected diagnosis of a deep-vein thrombosis, *pulmonary embolism* or both. Cases were matched with two controls by five year age-groups, districts of admission and date of admission. The controls were recruited from among women who were admitted to the hospitals with a diagnosis not associated with HRT. All the women were assessed for medical history, past and present HRT, past and present use of oral contraceptives, medications, height and weight, smoking and alcohol consumption and occupation. Women were excluded from the study if they had a history of pulmonary embolism, stroke or heart problems, recent surgery, cancer, long-term illness or pregnancy, and use of anticoagulants or oral contraceptives.

▶ **Espeland M, Applegate W, Furberg C, Lefkowitz D, Rice L, and Hunninghake D.**

Estrogen replacement therapy and progression of intimal-medial thickness in the carotid arteries of postmenopausal women. *American Journal of Epidemiology*, November 1995; 142:1011–1019. **Type:** Experimental (clinical trial)

Focus: The researchers examined the effect of hormone replacement therapy on three year changes in the carotid intimal-medial thickness. This study is one part of the Asymptomatic Carotid Atherosclerotic Progression Study (ACAPS).

Conclusions: HRT may reduce or halt the progression of early atherosclerosis in women not receiving active lipid-lowering medication. However, HRT did not affect *intimal-medial carotid* thickness in women assigned to Lovastatin.

Findings:

- Women who received Lovastatin, a lipid lowering medication, experienced a noticeable drop in LDL cholesterol.
- Intimal-medial carotid thickness in the placebo group increased in women who had not used HRT, but decreased in women who had used HRT.
- Lovastatin was associated with a 25 percent reduction in *low density lipoprotein cholesterol* among both HRT users and nonusers.
- HRT had a minimal effect in the intimal-medial carotid thickness in women receiving Lovastatin.
- Intimal-medial carotid thickness was identical among HRT users and nonusers of Warfarin.

Researchers' Comments: "Information of the specific type, route, or dose of estrogen was not collected in a standardized fashion; neither were data related to use of progestational agents" (1012).

Participants and Methods: Researchers collected ultrasonographic measurements of the carotid intimal-medial thickness from 1989 to 1993 in the Asymptomatic Carotid Artery Progression Study (ACAPS), which were compared with the intimal-medial thickness progression in women grouped according to HRT use. ACAPS a randomized, controlled clinical trial, assessed the impact of Lovastatin and Warfarin, both alone and in combination, on the development of carotid wall intimal-medial thickness in 919 asymptomatic women and men. The ACAPS' subjects were ages 40 to 79 years, had serum low density lipoprotein cholesterol between 160 and 189 mg/dl and had at least one other coronary risk factor. These subjects also had intimal-medial thickness of the carotid artery that showed atherosclerosis. The participants in this part of the ACAPS study were 186 postmenopausal women. These women were randomized and received either a placebo or Lovastatin with a placebo or Warfarin. The women were assessed for menopausal status and nonspecifically for HRT use. They were divided into three groups: current users of HRT at baseline, new users during the trial (no use of hormones two weeks before their baseline exam) and never users. Baseline HRT users were more likely to have had a hysterectomy than either new or nonusers and had a greater number of pregnancies, and more favorable baseline cholesterol values. Users and nonusers were similar in baseline blood pressure, body mass indexes, cross-sectional intimal-medial thickness of the carotid artery.

➤ **Gilabert J, Estelles A, Cano A, Espana F, Burrachina R, Grancha S, Aznar J, and Tortajada M.**

The effect of estrogen replacement therapy with or without progestogen on the fibrinolytic system and coagulation inhibitors in postmenopausal status. *American Journal of Obstetrics and Gynecology*, December 1995; 173:1849–1854. **Type:** Experimental (clinical trial)

Focus: The researchers analyzed several fibrinolytic components, coagulation inhibitors and lipid profile in postmenopausal women and evaluated the effects of HRT.

Conclusions: The increase in *fibrinolytic* activity and the decrease in *lipoprotein (a)* levels measured in women receiving HRT could help lower the risk of coronary heart disease associated with postmenopause. Many postmenopausal women exhibit lower fibrinolytic activity and an increase in lipoprotein (a) levels. An increase in lipoprotein (a) and a decrease in fribrinolytic activity can contribute to a increased risk of coronary heart disease after menopause.

Findings:
• The levels of lipoprotein (a) were significantly increased after menopause.
• Postmenopausal women who used HRT showed increased fibrinolytic activity.
• No significant modification in the levels of total cholesterol, triglycerides and glucose were observed in women who had undergone HRT.
• Women who received combined therapy (oral estrogen + progestogen) had a larger decrease in lipoprotein (a) levels than women who used transdermal estrogen, combined or alone.

Researchers' Comments: "The increase in lipoprotein (a) and the decrease in fibrinolytic activity can contribute to the increased risk of coronary disease after menopause" (1852).

Participants and Methods: Between October 1992 and October 1993, seventy-five postmenopausal (37 to 64 years) were enrolled in the clinical group. None of the women had any hormonal preparation during the eight weeks before the study. The women were screened to eliminate the possibility of confounding conditions such as endocrinologic and gastrointestinal disease. The control group consisted of nonmenopausal women ages 35 to 48 years who had not undergone HRT, and the experimental group were women of similar age who were given HRT. One group received oral estrogen plus progesterone and another group received transdermal estradiol plus progesterone. The final group received transdermal estradiol. Blood assays were performed in the 75 postmenopausal women before and after therapy.

➤ **Grady D, Herrington D, Bittner V, Blumenthal R, Davidson M, Hlatky M, Hsia J, Hulley S, Herd A, Khan S, Newby L, Waters D, Vittinghoff E, and Wenger N (for the HERS Research Group).**

Cardiovascular disease outcomes during 6.8 years of hormone therapy: Heart and Estrogen/Progestin Replacement Study follow-up (HERS II). *Journal of the American Medical Association*, July 2002; 288: 49–57. **Type:** Experimental (clinical trial)

Focus: An investigation to determine if the apparent decrease in the risk of a cardiovascular event observed in the later years of the HERS trial lasted through the HERS II study.

Conclusions: Women who used HRT in the follow-up period of the HERS study did not have a reduced risk of cardiovascular events. HRT should not be used in postmenopausal women to treat heart disease.

Findings:

• After 6.8 years, HRT (estrogen plus progestin) did not reduce the risk of cardiovascular events in women with diagnosed heart disease.

• Women who received combined therapy (estrogen plus progestin) did not have a reduced risk of cardiovascular events compared with those women who received the placebo.

• In 2.7 years of additional follow-up from the HERS study, no observed cardiovascular benefit in the HRT group although half the women continued to take the original assigned therapy.

• The decreased risk of cardiovascular events observed in the first HERS study at years three and five may have been a result of chance.

Researchers' Comments: "Our findings lend additional support to recent recommendations that postmenopausal hormone therapy should not be used for the purpose of reducing risk of CHD event in women with CHD" (57).

Participants and Methods: Participants in the first HERS study were 2763 postmenopausal women (average age 67 years) with a history of heart disease. The study was a blinded clinical trial in which women were randomized to receive 0.625 mg/d of conjugated estrogens plus 2.5 mg of medroxyprogesterone acetate or placebo. The women were assessed for medical conditions, cardiovascular status, estrogen use, blood chemistry, medications and reproductive history. The trial ended in 1998 and the participants were informed of their therapy assignment and the results of the initial trial. Participants who had received the placebo were advised not to start HRT for the prevention of Heart disease or cardiovascular events. Participants assigned the HRT were advised that it might be appropriate to continue HRT because there was some evidence that CHD event risk was reduced during years three and five. HERS II provided data from the cohort for an additional 2.7 years of follow-up conducted at outpatient and community setting at 20 U.S. clinical centers.

▶ **Grodstein F, Stampfer M, Manson J, Colditz G, Willett W, Rosner B, Speizer F, and Hennekens C.**

Postmenopausal estrogen and progestin use and the risk of cardiovascular disease. *The New England Journal of Medicine*, August 1996; 335:453–461. **Type:** Observational (cohort)

Focus: An examination of the relationship between cardiovascular disease and HRT.

Conclusions: Combined therapy (estrogen + progestin) does not have less of a cardioprotective effect than estrogen alone. Women who received combined therapy had a lower risk of cardiovascular disease than nonusers.

Findings:
• Women who used oral conjugated estrogen alone had a lower risk of heart disease than nonusers (**relative risk:** 0.60 for users/1.00 for nonusers).
• A increased risk for stroke was associated with HRT (**relative risk:** 1.27 for estrogen alone/1.09 for estrogen + progestin/1.00 for nonusers).
• A decreased risk of coronary heart disease was found in women who received estrogen + progestin as compared with nonusers.
• An increased risk of a stroke was found for women who used estrogen alone and this risk increased with a higher dosage (**relative risk:** 1.24 for users of 0.625 dosage/1.44 for users of 1.25 dosage).
• The benefit of HRT decreased after treatment was stopped.

Researchers' Comments: "Women who take hormones are a self-selected group and usually have healthier lifestyles with fewer risk factors than women who do not take hormones. In general-population samples, hormone users, as compared with nonusers, are leaner, drink more alcohol and participate in sports more often, even before starting hormones. However, these characteristics are due primarily to socioeconomic factors, since women who take hormones can generally afford medical care" (458).

Participants and Methods: The information in this study is based on the researches' analysis of 16 years of the follow-up data from the Nurses' Health Study which was initiated in 1976. Female nurses, age 30 to 55 years completed mailed questionnaires assessing their postmenopausal use of HRT and medical history. The data was updated every two years with follow-up questionnaires. Beginning in 1980, questions pertaining to diet and physical exercise were included and the women were also asked about the dose of conjugated estrogen. Follow-up occurred from 1976 to 1991.

➤ **Gruchow H, Anderson A, Barboriak J, and Sobocinski K.**

Postmenopausal use of estrogen and occlusion of coronary arteries. *American Heart Journal*, May 1988; 115:954–962. **Type:** Observational (case-control)

Focus: An assessment of the relationship between postmenopausal estrogen use and *coronary artery occlusion* in HRT users and nonusers.

Conclusion: Women who used HRT had a significant lower incidence of coronary artery occlusion. The effect of estrogen may be to reduce the risk of coronary heart disease by raising HDL cholesterol levels.

Findings:

• Postmenopausal women who received HRT had a lower incidence of coronary occlusion than nonusers (**odds ratio:** 0.59 (moderate occlusion) for users; 0.37 (severe occlusion) for users/ 1.00 for non-users).

• Total cholesterol and HDL cholesterol were the most important predictors of occlusion.

• Age at the time of *angiography*, postmenopausal estrogen use and plasma triglyceride level were also independent predictors of coronary artery occlusion.

• Women who received HRT used other drugs and medications (antacids, thyroid medication, tranquilizers, sedatives) more than nonusers; however, these medications did not affect the incidence of coronary occlusion.

• Estrogen users were more likely to have a lower body mass index and to exercise more.

Researchers' Comments: "Angiographically determined coronary occlusion assesses CHD more directly than symptoms (e.g., anginal pain) or mortality data. The most important disadvantage of using this outcome measure is the selective nature of patients who undergo arteriography" (961).

Participants and Methods: The researches selected participants from the Milwaukee Cardiovascular Data Registry that has data on 14,000 patients collected since 1968. From the registry, 933 postmenopausal women (50 to 75 years) were chosen as subjects. Of the study group, 154 estrogen users were younger than the 799 were nonusers (control group). These women had been referred for angiography in two Milwaukee hospitals between 1972 and 1985. The women were referred because of *angina*, *dyspnea* or recurrent chest pain. Angiograms were evaluated by an experienced cardiologist, and coronary occlusions were rated with a scoring range for zero to 300. The women were assessed using questionnaires for general medical history, family medical history, estrogen use, medicine use, lifestyle (exercise, alcohol intake, smoking), reproductive history and education. Fasting blood samples were obtained to measure cholesterol and triglyceride levels. Total cholesterol and triglyceride levels were obtained for the entire study population.

➤ Gutthann S, Rodriguez L, Castellsague J, and Oliart A.

Hormone replacement therapy and risk of venous thromboembolism: population based case-control study. *British Medical Journal*, March 1997; 314:796–800. **Type:** Observational (case-control)

Focus: An evaluation of the association between HRT and risk of venous thromboembolism.

Conclusions: *Venous thromboembolism* is associated with current use of HRT. However, the risk drops after the first year of use.

Findings:
- Women who were current users of HRT had an increased risk of venous thromboembolism (**odds ratio:** 2.10 for users/1.00 for nonusers)
- Women who used HRT had an elevated risk of venous thromboembolism in the first year of treatment (**odds ratio:** 4.60 for the first six months/3.00 for 6–12 months for users/1.00 for nonusers).
- Women who had a history of varicose veins, *phlebitis, bilateral oophorectomy* or obesity had a higher risk of thromboembolism.
- Past use of HRT was associated with a slight increased risk of thromboembolism (**odds ratio:** 1.40 for users/1.00 for nonusers).
- No differences in risk were found between different dosages and types of therapy (estrogen alone or combined), or types of preparations (oral & transdermal).

Researchers' Comments: "In a recent study, users of hormone replacement therapy had a better premenopausal cardiovascular risk factor profile than non-users. This type of bias, if present in our study, would underestimate the risk of venous thromboembolism among users of hormone replacement therapy" (799).

Participants and Methods: The study cohort involved 347,253 women (50 to 79 years) registered in the General Practice Research Database in the United Kingdom from January 1991 to October 1994. Women who had a history of thromboembolic events or other risk factors were excluded from the study. The cases were 292 women admitted to the hospital for a first onset of *pulmonary embolism* or venous thromboembolism. The control group consisted of 10,000 women randomly selected from the original study group. All participants were assessed for general health, medical conditions, reproductive history, medications and HRT (type, dosage, duration).

➤ Haines C, Chung T, Chang A, Masarei J, Tomlinson B, and Wong E.

Effect of oral estradiol on Lp(a) and other lipoproteins in postmenopausal women. *Archives of Internal Medicine,* April 1996; 156:866–872. **Type:** Experimental (clinical trial)

Focus: An investigation of the effectiveness of HRT in lowering the concentration of Lp(a) in postmenopausal women who had undergone hysterectomies.

Conclusions: Oral estradiol reduced lipoprotein (a) levels in the bloodstream. HRT may have a protective effect on the heart in postmenopausal women by lowering Lp(a) levels.

Findings:
• Lipoprotein (a) levels were reduced in women receiving HRT compared with the placebo group.
• Higher concentrations of lipoprotein (a) were associated with higher levels of total cholesterol and LDL cholesterol.
• Women who received HRT had a reduction in total cholesterol and LDL cholesterol.
• Women who received HRT had an increase in triglyceride levels.

Researchers' Comments: "The magnitude of the reduction of Lp(a) lipoprotein levels was not as great as has been demonstrated with niacin.... A larger study would be useful to determine whether the reduction in Lp(a) lipoprotein concentrations became significant with long-term estrogen use" (872).

Participants and Methods: The participants were 100 postmenopausal women who had undergone hysterectomies. This trial was a double-blind, placebo-controlled, crossover study conducted for a year. The women were recruited from the Hormone Replacement Clinic of the Department of Obstetrics and Gynecology, Prince of Wales Hospital, in Hong Kong. The women were randomize into one to two groups. Group one women received 2 mg of oral estradiol daily for the first six months and placebo for the second six months. Group two received placebo for the first six months, and 2 mg of daily oral estradiol for the second six months. Blood was drawn and analyzed from the women before the study began, at the time of the sixth month crossover and at the completion of the treatment. The following plasma constituents were analyzed and measured: total cholesterol, high density lipoprotein cholesterol, low-density lipoprotein cholesterol, triglycerides, HDL subfractions, apolipoprotein (apo) A-I and apo B and lipoprotein (a). To assess the long-term effect of estradiol on Lp(a) levels at the completion of the crossover study, all available subjects from other groups were treated with the same dose of estradiol for a longer period of twelve months. Samples were taken at the end of treatment and compared with values at the completion of the crossover study.

➤ **Hassager C, Riis B, Strom V, Guyene T, and Christiansen C.**

The long-term effect of oral and percutaneous estradiol on plasma renin substrate and blood pressure. **Circulation,** October 1987; 76:753–758. **Type:** Experimental (clinical trial)

Focus: An examination of the effect of HRT on blood pressure, plasma renin substrate and serum estrogens.

Conclusions: HRT (oral and *percutaneous* estradiol) may protect postmenopausal from an increase in diastolic blood pressure associated with aging.

Findings:
- *Diastolic blood pressure* decreased in women who received HRT (oral and transdermal).
- Women who received HRT (oral estradiol) had an increase in *plasma renin substrate* levels after 12 months of treatment.
- Women who received HRT (transdermal) did not have an increase in plasma renin substrate.
- *Systolic blood pressure* was not changed with HRT.
- The addition of progestin did not have an effect on estradiol levels, blood pressure or renin substrate.

Researchers' Comments: "The increase in plasma renin substrate observed in the oral estradiol group might, theoretically, cause development of hypertension. However, no significant correlation was found between plasma renin substrate and systolic or diastolic blood pressure in any of the groups" (757).

Participants and Methods: The study was part of a double-blind clinical trial carried out in a hospital setting in Glostrup, Denmark from June 1983 to December 1985. The study involved 110 postmenopausal women who completed the trial. The women were assessed for general and reproductive health, blood pressure and blood chemistry. Women were excluded if they had any indication or history of conditions which influenced calcium or liver metabolism. The women were assigned to one of four treatment groups: oral cyclical combined therapy (2 mg estradiol valerate + cyproterone acetate), oral placebo, percutaneous estradiol supplemented by 200 mg oral progestin during the second year, and percutaneous placebo cream. At baseline and at various points throughout the study, the women were assessed for systolic and diastolic blood pressure, body weight, blood lipid levels, serum estrone and estradiol levels. Plasma renin substrate levels were measured at baseline, year one and year two.

➤ **Heckbert S, Kaplan R, Weiss N, Psaty B, Lin D, Furberg C, Starr J, Anderson G, and LaCroix A.**

Risk of recurrent coronary events in relation to use and recent initiation of postmenopausal hormone therapy. ***Archives Internal Medicine***, July 2001; 161:1709–1713. **Type:** Observational (cohort)

Focus: An examination of the risk of coronary events (heart attacks or coronary related death) in women who use HRT with established heart disease.

Conclusions: The results from this study support the HERS study, suggesting an increased risk in coronary events in women with heart disease after starting HRT.

Findings:

• Women with established heart disease had an increased risk of heart attack especially within the first 60 days after starting HRT (***relative hazard:*** 2.16 for users/1.00 for nonusers).

• Women who used HRT and survived after a first coronary event had no overall difference in risk of a recurrent coronary event than nonusers (***relative hazard:*** 0.96 for users/1.00 for nonusers).

- After one year women who used HRT had a reduced risk of a coronary event even with a history of heart disease (*relative hazard:* 0.76 for users/1.00 for nonusers).

Researchers Comments: "At present, the only clinical trial data available suggest no beneficial effect of hormone therapy in women with established CHD and the possibility of an early increase in risk after starting hormone therapy" (1713).

Participants Methods: The participants, 981 postmenopausal women, were drawn from the Group Health Cooperative, a health maintenance organization. These women had survived a coronary event between July 1986 and December 1996. A pharmacy database provided information about hormone use and coronary events were obtained from medical records. The women were assessed for general health, estrogen use, medical conditions, blood chemistry, smoking history, and weight. Hormone replacement therapies included estrogen alone or estrogen plus progestin. The most commonly used estrogens were conjugated and esterified. Unopposed estrogen was used 67 percent of the time and estrogen plus progestin was used 33 percent of the time.

> **Hulley S, Grady D, Bush T, Furberg C, Herrington D, Riggs B, and Vittinghoff E (for the Heart and Estrogen/Progestin Replacement Study (HERS) Research Group).**

Randomized trial of estrogen plus progestin for secondary prevention of coronary heart disease in postmenopausal women. *Journal of the American Medical Association*, August 1998; 280:605–613. **Type:** Experimental (clinical trial)

Focus: An investigation of HRT (combined therapy) and the risk of coronary heart disease in postmenopausal women with a known history of coronary heart disease.

Conclusions: Combined therapy (estrogen + progestin) did not reduce the number of *coronary events* in postmenopausal women with known heart disease during a 4-year follow-up period. Women who received HRT (combined therapy) had an increase incidence of thromboembolism and gallbladder disease.

Findings:
- Women who received combined therapy (conjugated equine estrogen + medroxyprogesterone acetate) had more coronary events than women who received a placebo.
- Women who received HRT (combined therapy) had a higher inci-

dence of thromboembolism (three times that of nonusers) and a higher incidence of gall bladder disease.

• Women who received HRT (combined therapy) had more cardiac events than the placebo group during the first year on HRT, but they had fewer events during the four and five years of HRT.

• The HRT group experienced 71 coronary heart disease deaths; the placebo group experienced 58 coronary heart disease deaths.

• In the HRT group, HDL cholesterol increased (8 percent), LDL cholesterol decreased (14 percent) and triglyceride levels increased (10 percent).

Researchers' Comments: "We do not recommend starting this treatment for the purpose of secondary prevention of CHD" (612).

Participants and Methods: The participants in this study were postmenopausal women recruited from January 1993 to September 1994 at twenty HERS clinical centers. In all, 2763 women enrolled in this double-blinded, randomized placebo-controlled clinical trial. The predominantly white study group ranged in age from 44 to 79 years. The HRT group had 1380 women and the placebo group had 1383 women. At baseline the women were assessed for general and reproductive health, medical history, reproductive history, risk factors for coronary heart disease, medications, demographic characteristics, lipoprotein cholesterol and triglyceride levels. Treatment consisted of conjugated equine estrogen (0.625 mg/daily) plus medroxyprogesterone acetate (2.5 mg/daily) or the placebo. The following conditions excluded women from the study: HRT within three months of the screening visits; a coronary heart event within the previous six months; elevated triglyceride levels; a history of a deep vein thrombosis or pulmonary embolism; a history of breast cancer; other gynecological cancers or conditions. Follow-up averaged about 4.1 years. A follow-up visit was scheduled every four months to assess compliance, provide medication and obtain data on outcome and adverse events.

▶ **Hulley S, Furberg C, Barrett-Connor E, Cauley J, Grady D, Haskell W, Knopp R, Lowery M, Satterfield S, Schrott H, Vittinghoff E, and Hunninghake D (for the HERS Research Group).**

Noncardiovascular disease outcomes during 6.8 years of hormone therapy (Heart and Estrogen/Progestin Replacement Study follow-up, HERS II). *Journal of the American Medical Association*, July 2002; 288: 58–66. **Type:** Experimental (clinical trial)

Focus: An examination of the relation between long-term HRT and the development of disease in postmenopausal women with known heart disease.

Conclusions: Women, with diagnosed coronary heart disease, who received combined therapy (estrogen + progestin) for a duration of 6.8 years, had an increased risk of venous thromboembolism and *biliary tract surgery*.

Findings:

- Women who received HRT (combined therapy) had an increased risk of venous thromboembolism with a relative hazard of 2.08 compared with 1.00 for nonusers.
- Women who received HRT (combined therapy) had an increased risk for biliary tract surgery (**relative hazard:** 1.48 for users/1.00 for nonusers).
- Women who received HRT (combined therapy) had a slight but not a significant increase in risk of breast cancer (**relative hazard:** 1.27 for users/1.00 for nonusers).
- Hip fractures increased for HRT users (**relative hazard:** 1.61 for users/1.00 for users).
- Death rates were higher in women who received HRT (combined therapy) 1.10 for users/1.00 for nonusers)

Researchers' Comments: "We recorded 261 deaths in the hormone group and 239 in the placebo group. The absence of mortality benefit contrasts with the finding in observations studies of lower mortality rates among women who use postmenopausal hormones compared with nonusers. Population differences could underlie this disparity, but we believe that the lower mortality rate among hormone users in observational studies is primarily due to confounding: women who seek hormone therapy and remain compliant tend to be healthier and wealthier than those who do not. Because these characteristics cannot be measured precisely, their influence cannot be adequately addressed by statistical adjustment in observational studies" (64).

Participants and Methods: Participants in this clinical trial (The Heart and Estrogen/Progestin Replacement Study, HERS) were 2,763 postmenopausal women (average age 67 years) with diagnosed heart disease. The trial was conducted between 1993 and 2000 at outpatient and community setting at twenty U.S. clinical centers. The study was randomized, blinded and placebo-controlled for 4.1 years (HERS) to investigate the effects of combined therapy in older women with coronary disease. HERS II became an observational follow-up study for disease surveillance for 2.7 more years. During HERS II many women randomized to hormones took open-label (unblinded) estrogen prescribed by their physicians but only a few of those assigned to placebo did. During baseline the women were assessed for general health, menopause status, medical conditions, medications, estrogen use and mammography. All baseline measures excluding demographics and health history were repeated at the final HERS visit, an average of four months before enrollment in HER II. During the HERS trial, women were randomly allocated to receive either 0.625 mg/daily of conjugated estrogen plus 2.5 mg of medroxyprogesterone acetate or an identical placebo. Information regarding disease events was obtained from hospital records, death certificates and follow-up information.

➤ **Jick H, Derby L, Myers M, Vasilakis C, Newton K.**

Risk of hospital admission for idiopathic venous thromboembolism among users of postmenopausal oestrogens. *The Lancet*, October 1996; 348:981–983. **Type:** Observational (case control)

Focus: An exploration of the relation between postmenopausal estrogen use and the occurrence of *idiopathic venous thromboembolism*.

Conclusions: Women who use HRT have a higher risk of venous thromboembolism than nonusers. The risk increased with increasing dosages of estrogen.

Findings:
* Current users of estrogen (0.625 mg/d) had an increased risk of venous thromboembolism (*relative risk estimate:* 3.30 for users/6.90 for users of 1.25 mg/daily/1.00 for nonusers).
* Current users of estrogen (0.325 mg/d) had an increased risk of venous thromboembolism (*relative risk estimate:* 2.10 for users/1.00 nonusers).
* Current users estrogen (1.25 mg/d) had an elevated risk of venous thromboembolism (*relative risk estimate:* 6.90 for users/1.00 nonusers).
* Year one of HRT posed the highest risk for users (*relative risk estimate:* 6.70 for users/1.00 for nonusers).
* Because idiopathic venous thromboembolism is rare, the increased risk did not contribute to excess *morbidity*.

Researchers Comments: "Current oestrogen users are three to four times more likely to have idiopathic VTE than non-users (982).

Participants Methods: This study was based on information gathered from the Group Health Cooperative of Puget Sound, Washington from 1980 to 1994. The cases were postmenopausal women (50 to 74 years)

who had been admitted to the hospital for idiopathic venous thromboembolism and were identified through hospital records. The cases were
matched to controls by age and duration of cooperative membership. All
the participants were assessed for general health, medical conditions, reproductive history, body-mass index, cigarette consumption, medication use
and HRT (type, dosage, duration). Women were excluded if they had been
admitted to the hospital for trauma or surgery within six months before
the embolism, or had any of the following conditions: epilepsy, stroke, cancer, kidney failure, diabetes, cardiovascular conditions.

➤ Kim C, Ryu W, Kwak J, Park C, and Ryoo U.

Changes in Lp(a) lipoprotein and lipid levels after cessation of female
sex hormone production and estrogen replacement therapy. *Archives of
Internal Medicine,* March 1996; 156:500–504. **Type:** Observational
(case-control)

Focus: An investigated the changes in Lp(a) lipoprotein cholesterol
levels in women who had a surgical menopause and who subsequently
received HRT.

Conclusions: Women who received HRT and who had a hysterectomy had lower Lp(a) levels and increased HDL (good cholesterol) levels.
HRT may be protective of the heart because it lowers Lp(a) levels.

Findings:

• Lp(a) lipoprotein levels were increase after *bilateral oophorectomy* but
  lowered with HRT.
• HDL levels were raised in the BSO group (*bilateral salpingo-oophorectomy)* of women who received HRT.
• After four months, LDL cholesterol levels in both groups increased at
  2 months and decreased almost to basal level at 4 months.
• Both groups of women (receiving HRT and no HRT) had increased
  triglyceride levels after hysterectomies.
• The USO group (non HRT) had an increase in Lp(a) lipoprotein cholesterol at two months but returned to basal level by four months.

Researchers' Comments: "In the BSO group, the HDL cholesterol level was not changed after two months. This finding implied that
menopause does not reduce the HDL cholesterol level, and this is inconsistent with the findings of previous reports" (503).

Participants and Methods: Forty-four premenopausal women
(30 to 53 years) who had undergone transdominal hysterectomies (TAH)
were the participants in this study. Two groups were created: women who
had a TAH and a unilateral salpingo-oophorectomy, and women who had

a bilateral salphingo-oophorectomy. Blood was sampled and analyzed before the operation and after the operation (2 months and 4 months). Lp(a) lipoprotein, total cholesterol, HDL cholesterol, LDL cholesterol, VLDL cholesterol and triglyceride were measured. HRT (0.625mg/conjugated estrogen) was given daily to the BSO group two months after the operation.

> **Koh K, Mincemoyer R, Bui M, Csako G, Pucino F, Guetta V, Waclawiw M, and Cannon R.**

Effects of hormone-replacement therapy on fibrinolysis in postmenopausal women. *The New England Journal of Medicine*, March 1997; 336:683–689. **Type:** Experimental (clinical trial)

Focus: An examination of the effects of HRT on fibrinolysis in postmenopausal women.

Conclusions: HRT (estrogen alone or combined therapy) reduces *PAI-1* levels in many postmenopausal women indicating an increase in *fibrinolysis*. However, transdermal HRT did not reduce PAI-1 levels or significantly alter cholesterol levels.

Findings:

- Oral HRT, estrogen alone or combined therapy (estrogen + progestin) reduced LDL cholesterol and increased HDL cholesterol.
- Oral HRT reduced PAI-1 levels; transdermal HRT did not.
- Transdermal estradiol, alone or in a combination with progestin (medroxyprogesterone acetate) did not increase HDL levels.
- Neither estradiol alone nor combined therapy (estradiol + progestin) caused any significant change in lipoproteins except for a slight decrease in total cholesterol with combined therapy.
- HRT (conjugated estrogen alone or combined therapy) reduced PAI-1 level by about 50 percent.

Researchers Comments: "Although significant reductions in PAI-1 levels were detected in our study after oral hormone-replacement therapy, some women had no change in PAI-1 ... this was especially true of those with relatively low pretreatment PAI-1 values. In these women, the procoagulant effects of therapy ... may negate much of the cardiovascular benefit of hormone therapy or even increase the risk of thromboembolic events (689).

Participants Method: Two groups of postmenopausal women participated in this study. The first group of 30 women (50–60 years) were randomly assigned to a treatment protocol for one month: 0.625 mg of oral conjugated estrogen daily or 0.625 mg of conjugated estrogen and 2.5 mg of medroxyprogesterone acetate daily. After one month washout period, each woman received the other therapy for one month. In the second group, 20 women were randomly assigned to begin one month of treatment with either 0.1 mg of transdermal estradiol daily or 0.1 mg of estradiol and 2.5 mg of medroxyprogesterone acetate daily, with a one month washout period before receiving the other therapy. None of the women had received antioxidant vitamins, cholesterol-lowering drugs, or estrogen two months before the study.

➤ **Manolio T, Furberg C, Shemanski L, Psaty B, O'Leary D, Tracy R, and Bush T (the CHS Collaborative Research Group)**

Association of postmenopausal estrogen use with cardiovascular disease and its risk factors in older women. *Circulation*, November 1993; 88:2163–2171. **Type:** Observational (cohort)

Focus: An investigation of the association of past and present HRT with cardiovascular risk factors.

Conclusions: Postmenopausal women who use HRT have a favorable cardiovascular profile and a lower measure of cardiovascular disease than nonusers.

Findings:

• Estrogen use past or present was associated with lower LDL cholesterol and higher HDL cholesterol.

• Estrogen users had fewer vascular conditions based on measurements of the *carotid artery* and other measurements).

• Estrogen users had lower levels of *glucose*, fibrinogen and *insulin*.

• Estrogen users were less inclined to be obese.

• Women who smoked and used estrogen were not significantly different from nonusers who smoked in risk factors and other conditions.

Researchers' Comments: "The lack of associations with duration of use probably reflected the unreliability of the duration data, which depended on recall of sometimes distant events and which were missing in a large proportion of estrogen users" (2169).

Participants and Methods: The findings from this study are a part of the Cardiovascular Health Study (CHS), a prospective study of the risk factors for coronary heart disease and stroke in 5201 men and women (65 or more years). Data was obtained from a number of centers and participants were randomly recruited from the Health Care Financing Administration Medicare eligibility list from four communities in the following states: North Carolina, California, Maryland and Pennsylvania. The sample included 2955 women (65 to 100 years) with the average age of 72.4 years. At baseline the participants were assessed for general health, medical conditions, medical history, medication usage, physical activity, reproductive history and HRT (type, dosage, duration). Measurements of the following were taken: cognitive functioning, blood pressure, weight, height, waist/hip circumference, body fat, blood chemistry, lung volume, carotid artery thickness, heart functioning. Of the 2955 women, 12 percent were using oral estrogen or combined therapy (estrogen + progestin). Also, 26 percent of the women reported past use of hormones. Estrogen users were younger, more likely to be white, had more education and income than nonusers. Furthermore, estrogen users had more prior hysterectomies than nonusers.

➤ Munk-Jensen N, Ulrich L, Obel E, Nielsen S, Edwards D, and Meinertz H.

Continuous combined and sequential estradiol and norethindrone acetate treatment of postmenopausal women. Effect on plasma lipoproteins in a two-year placebo-controlled trial. *American Journal of Obstetrics and Gynecology*, July 1994; 171:132–138. **Type:** Experimental (clinical trial)

Focus: An examination of the effects of HRT (combined therapy) on plasma lipoprotein levels.

Conclusions: Combined therapy (estrogen + progestin) lowered total cholesterol and LDL cholesterol. Continuous combined therapy, however, reduced HDL cholesterol. The addition of progestin (*norethindrone acetate*) for the purpose of preventing *endometrial hyperplasia* reduces the increased HDL cholesterol found when estrogen is administered alone.

Findings:

• Women receiving HRT in the form of combined therapy had a decrease in LDL cholesterol and total cholesterol.

• The placebo group (no HRT) had no change in plasma lipid or lipoprotein levels.

• Women who received *sequential combined therapy* had an increase in triglyceride levels.

• Women who received *continuous combined therapy* had a significant decrease in HDL cholesterol.

• Women who received sequential combined therapy did not have a decrease in HDL cholesterol.

Researchers' Comments: "Because estrogen monotherapy may reduce cardiovascular risk of postmenopausal women, possibly in part by elevating HDL cholesterol and decreasing LDL levels, the observed effects of combined treatment require careful evaluation of the roles of LDL and HDL in coronary heart disease" (136).

Participants and Methods: The study involved postmenopausal women (51 to 53 years) residing in Frederiksborg, Denmark. Women were excluded from the study if they had a history of breast cancer, endometrial cancer, thromboembolic disease, liver disease, chronic pancreatitis, diabetes and a number of other conditions. The final study group from which data was obtained consisted of 113 subjects. Baseline values of blood lipids and lipoproteins were assessed. The women were also given a gynecological exam and a blood pressure was measured. The women were randomized into one of three treatment groups. Group A received continuous combined therapy (2 mg estradiol + 1 mg norethindrone acetate). Group B received sequential combined therapy (2 mg estradiol for 12 days and 2 mg estradiol and 1mg norethindrone acetate for the following 10 days and 1 mg of estradiol for the final 6 days). Group C, the control group, received a placebo. Blood was drawn at the twenty-fourth cycle during the progestogen phase of the cycle to determine blood lipids and lipoprotein levels.

➤ **Nabulsi A, Folsom A, White A, Patsch W, Heiss G, Wu K, and Szklo M.**

Association of hormone-replacement with various cardiovascular risk factors in postmenopausal women. *The New England Journal of Medicine*, April 1993; 328:1069–1075. **Type:** Observational (*cross-sectional study*)

Focus: An investigation of the association of HRT (estrogen alone or combined) and cardiovascular risk.

Conclusions: HRT is associated with a positive physiologic profile that may provide protection against cardiovascular disease.

Findings:
• Current users of HRT had higher HDL cholesterol than nonusers.
• Current uses of HRT had lower levels of LDL cholesterol than nonusers.
• Current users of HRT had lower levels of lipoprotein (a) and *fibrinogen.*
• Current users of HRT had lower fasting glucose levels and insulin levels than nonusers.
• Current users of HRT (estrogen alone) had higher triglyceride levels, factor VII and Protein C levels than nonusers or women who used combined therapy.

Researchers' Comments: "Because our study was not a randomized trial, we cannot rule out selection bias related to hormone replacement or certain other noncausal explanations of the findings. Nevertheless, it is of interest to estimate the potential effect of these physiologic findings, if causal, on the risk of coronary heart disease" (1074).

Participants and Methods: This cross-sectional analysis used data from the Atherosclerosis Risk in Communities study (1986–1989) involving 15,800 subjects from four population samples of men and women (45 to 64 years) in North Carolina, Mississippi, Minneapolis and Maryland. The final study group consisted of 4958 postmenopausal women. The participants were assessed for blood chemistry, general health, alcohol and cigarette consumption, medical conditions, reproductive history, medication use, carotid artery status, physical activity and other demographics. Postmenopausal women (4958) with no cardiovascular disease at baseline formed the study group. These women were assigned to one of four groups: current users of estrogen alone, current users of estrogen plus progestin, nonusers who formerly used hormones and never users of HRT. Only 21 percent of the women in the study were currently using HRT and conjugated equine estrogen (Premarin) was used by 83 percent of these women. Combined therapy (estrogen + progestin) was used by 17 percent of the current users of HRT.

> **Ottosson U, Johansson B, and von Schoultz B.**

Subfractions of high-density lipoprotein cholesterol during estrogen replacement therapy: a comparison between progestogens and natural progesterone. *Journal of Obstetrics and Gynecology*, March 1985; 151: 746–750. **Type:** Experimental (clinical trial)

Focus: An investigation of the effects of *progestogens* compared with *natural progesterone* on HDL cholesterol and apolipoproteins.

Conclusions: Progestogens reduced HDL cholesterol in the women using HRT. Natural progesterone did not affect HDL cholesterol levels in women who used it for HRT.

Findings:
- All the women who were treated with *estradiol valerate* and synthetic progestogens had withdrawal bleeding during the week off of treatment.
- Women who had sequential progestogen *(levonorgestrel or medroxyprogesterone acetate)* as part of combined cyclic therapy, had a drop in HDL cholesterol about 18 percent and 28 percent after one cycle.
- Estrogen therapy (estradiol valerate, 2 mg) increased HDL cholesterol levels and the concentration of *apolipoproteins.*
- Women who received natural micronized progesterone (100mg) did not have a change in HDL cholesterol or apolipoproteins.

- Ten women who took natural progesterone had regular withdrawal bleeding and no side affects such as weight gain or mood change.

Researchers' Comments: "Micronized progesterone may develop into an attractive alternative to synthetic progestogens in clinical practice" (750).

Participants and Methods: The participants were 58 women (46–69 years) who had attended a clinic in Sweden because of menopausal symptoms. HRT involved cyclic treatment of unopposed estrogen (estradiol valerate) 2 mg daily for a duration of three cycles. After the third cycle the women were randomly assigned to one of three groups for the addition of either progestogens (levonorgestrel or medroxyprogesterone acetate) or natural micronized progesterone. These hormones were given the last 10 days of each treatment cycle. Twenty women received 250 μg of levonorgestrel daily. Twenty women received 5 mg of medroxyprogesterone acetate twice daily, and 18 women were given 100 mg of micronized progesterone twice daily. Blood was drawn and analyzed for lipoprotein levels before and during therapy.

> **Perrone G, Stefanutti C, Galoppi P, Anelli G, Capri O, Lucani G, Vivenzio A, Mazzarella B, and Zichella L.**

Effect of oral and transdermal hormone replacement therapy on lipid profile and LP(a) level in menopausal women with hypercholesterolemia. *International Journal of Fertility*, Nov.–Dec. 1996; 41:509–515.
Type: Experimental (clinical trial)

Focus: An evaluation of the effect of HRT on plasma lipoproteins in forty-two postmenopausal women with high cholesterol (*hypercholesterolemia*).

Conclusions: Transdermal estrogen and oral estrogens combined with progestin have a positive outcome on total cholesterol and LDL cholesterol. However, HRT did not alter Lp(a) levels in women receiving treatment.

Findings:
- After six months, women who received combined therapy (transdermal estrogen or oral estrogen plus progestin) had a decrease in total cholesterol and HDL cholesterol.
- Lp(a) levels were not changed by HRT.
- At six months, both HRT groups (transdermal estrogen + progestin and oral estrogen + progestin) had an increase in triglycerides.
- The ratio of HDL cholesterol to LDL cholesterol was improved in the HRT groups, but not in the control group in which it decreased.

• After six months both HRT groups had a reduction in total cholesterol: transdermal estrogen + progestin users (–11.5 percent) and oral estrogen + progestin users (–11.3 percent).

Researchers' Comments: "No significant changes in Lp(a) levels were observed in any patients after 3 or 6 months of treatment" (512).

Participants and Methods: This randomized small Italian study involved forty-two menopausal women, sixty years or less, who were diagnosed with hypercholesterolemia, cholesterol greater than 240 mg/dl. The women participating in the study were assessed for general health, medical conditions, medications, blood chemistry and hormone use. Before the study began, the women were required to stop any medical treatment that would interfere or affect their serum lipid levels. The participants were assigned to one of three treatment groups: transdermal estradiol plus progestin (50 μg twice a week given continuously plus medroxyprogesterone acetate 10 mg/d for 12 days each month), conjugated equine estrogens plus progestin (0.625 mg/d–Premarin given continuously plus medroxyprogesterone acetate 10 mg/d for 12 days each month), and the control group that did not receive treatment. Fourteen women were in the transdermal plus progestin group and fourteen women were in the oral estrogen plus progestin group. Three women were in the control group. Blood analysis was performed at baseline and again at three months and six months. Total cholesterol, HDL cholesterol, LDL cholesterol, Lp(a) levels and triglycerides were measured as part of the blood chemistry analysis. Five women did not complete the study leaving before the third month for various reasons.

➤ **Pradhan A, Manson J, Rossouw J, Siscovick D, Mouton C, Rifai N, Wallace R, Jackson R, Pettinger M, and Ridker P.**

Inflammatory biomarkers hormone replacement therapy, and incident coronary heart disease: prospective analysis from the Women's Health Initiative observational study. *Journal of the American Medical Association*, August 2002; 288:980–987. **Type:** Observational (case-control within a cohort study)

Focus: An investigation with two purposes: an examination of the relationship between blood levels of the inflammatory biomarkers (*C-reactive protein* and *interleukin* 6) and the development of coronary heart diseases; the assessment of the relationship between HRT, inflammatory biomarkers and the development of coronary heart disease.

Conclusions: Higher blood levels of inflammatory biomarkers (e.g.,

C-reactive protein and interleukin 6) are strong predictors of adverse cardiovascular events in postmenopausal women despite HRT status.

Findings:

- Higher blood levels of inflammatory biomarkers are independent factors increasing the risk of an adverse cardiac event.
- Women who used HRT (estrogen) had higher levels of C-reactive protein, but not interleukin 6 (IL-6).
- Plasma concentrations of CRP and IL-6 were higher among cases than among controls within each category of HRT use.
- CRP values were 55 percent higher in cases who were current users of HRT compared with cases who were nonusers of HRT.
- C-reactive proteins and interleukin 6 were both associated with an increased risk of an adverse cardiac event
- Women who had the same baseline levels of inflammatory biomarkers had a twofold increased risk for developing coronary heart disease whether they were users or nonusers of HRT.

Researchers' Comments: "That use or nonuse of HRT had less importance than expressed CRP levels in terms of cardiovascular risk assessment also implies that diet, exercise, and smoking cessation are likely to remain the most important interventions for the primary prevention of vascular disease for some time to come" (987).

Participants and Methods: The Women's Health Initiative cohort study, with a clinical trial and observational study arm, was initiated in 1994 involving more than 75,000 postmenopausal women (50 to 79 years) who participated in the trial at 40 clinical centers in the United States. The participants were assessed for general health, medical conditions, estrogen use, reproductive status, medications, blood pressure, and blood chemistry (HDL cholesterol, LDL cholesterol, C-reactive proteins, interleukin 6, and triglycerides). Eighty-two percent of the current users were taking oral conjugated equine estrogens, and 74 percent were treated with a dose of 6.25 mg/daily. Eighty-seven percent of current users HRT (combined therapy) were taking estrogen with medroxyprogesterone acetate, (2.5, 5.0 or 10 mg/daily). Follow-up was approximately every 2.9 years. The participants received medical questionnaires and researchers reviewed medical records, death certificates and autopsy reports. This prospective nested case-control study analyzed 304 cases of women participating in the WHI who developed coronary artery disease and matched them with controls who were free of coronary heart disease and cancer. Cases and controls were similar in age, smoking status, ethnicity, and follow-up time.

➤ **Psaty B, Smith N, Lemaitre R,
Heckbert S, LaCroix A, Rosendaal F.**

Hormone replacement therapy, prothrombotic mutations, and the risk of incident nonfatal myocardial infarction in postmenopausal women. *Journal of the American Medical Association*, February 2001; 285: 906–912. **Type:** Observational (case control)

Focus: An investigation of the effect of *prothrombotic mutations* on the incidence of heart attacks.

Conclusions: Women who are postmenopausal, have high blood pressure and prothrombotic mutations have a higher risk of heart attack than women without the mutation.

Findings:

• Women with high blood pressure and the prothrombotic mutation who used HRT had an elevated risk of heart attack (odds ratio: 20.7 for users/1.00 nonusers).

• Women with high blood pressure and the prothrombotic mutation who were not users of HRT had only a very slight increased risk of heart attack (odds ratio: 1.15/1.00 users for non users with prothrombotic mutation).

• Women without high blood pressure who used HRT and had the prothrombotic mutation had a slight increased risk of heart attack (odds ratio: 1.24 for users/1.00 for nonusers with prothrombotic mutation).

Researchers Comments: "The findings of this study suggest the possibility of an interaction between the prothrombin variant and HRT use on the incidence of MI among women with hypertension.... (912)

Participants and Methods: Participants in this study were enrolled in the Group Health Cooperative (GHC), a Seattle, Washington, based health maintenance organization. The cases were 232 postmenopausal women (30–79 years) who had survived a heart attack between January 1995 and December 1998. The controls, 723 postmenopausal women, were a stratified and randomized sample of women with no history of heart attack. Cases and controls were matched by age, calendar year and *hypertension* status using outpatient medical records, telephone interviews and lab data. The women were assessed for general health, medical conditions, heart disease risk factors, estrogen use, menopausal status, and prothrombotic mutation status. Esterified estrogens were the most frequently used form of estrogen for HRT in this study group.

➤ **Shemesh J, Frenkel Y, Leibovitch L, Grossman E, Pines A, Motro M.**

Does hormone replacement therapy inhibit coronary artery calcification? *Obstetrics and Gynecology*, June 1997; 89:989–992. **Type:** Experimental (clinical trial)

Focus: An investigation to assess the relationship between HRT and the calcification of arteries in postmenopausal women using double helical computed tomography (CT).

Conclusions: HRT reduces the prevalence of *coronary calcification* in postmenopausal women.

Findings:

• Coronary calcification was found in 28.2 percent of the women.
• Women who did not use HRT (the control group) had a higher prevalence of coronary calcification than users.
• Coronary calcification was 14.6 percent for users of HRT and 43.2 percent for nonusers of HRT.
• Age and coronary risk factors were not important in determining coronary calcification but HRT was an important determinant.

Researchers' Comments: "The different rate of coronary calcium suggests a difference in the development of atherosclerosis. We found coronary calcium in 28.2 percent of the women studied...." (991)

Participants and Methods: Postmenopausal women were recruited from a postmenopausal outpatient clinic. Seventy-eight women, averaging 57 years old, underwent CT scanning to assess the extent of coronary calcification. Forty-one women were HRT users and had been so for at least four years. The control group, thirty-seven nonusers of HRT, were age-matches with the other subjects. The participants were assessed for FSH levels, estradiol blood sugar, serum cholesterol levels and risk factors for coronary heart disease. Women were excluded from the study if they had a surgical menopause or any indication of a history of coronary artery disease. Both groups had some women with the following health related conditions: smoking, hypertension, family history, hypercholesterolemia and diabetes. Nonusers had a higher incidence diabetes. HRT users received conjugated estrogen (0.625 mg/d) plus medroxyprogesterone acetate (5 mg). The estrogen was taken every day and the progestin on days 13–25 of each month.

➤ **Snabes M, Payne J, Kopelen H, Dunn J, Young R, and Zoghbi W.**

Physiologic estradiol replacement therapy and cardiac structure and function in normal postmenopausal women: a randomized, double-blind, placebo-controlled, crossover trial. *Obstetrics and Gynecology,* March 1997; 89:332–339. **Type:** Experimental (Clinical Trial)

Focus: An investigation of the effect of estradiol (HRT) on cardiac structure and function in postmenopausal women.

Conclusions: HRT (*estradiol*) does not affect cardiac structure or function in postmenopausal women. This study does not support the idea that HRT (estradiol) improves cardiovascular function.

Findings:
• Heart rate, *systolic and diastolic* pressures were unchanged after three months of treatment.
• None of the treatment parameters showed any change after three months of estradiol HRT.

Researchers' Comments: "These findings corroborate earlier experimental data showing no significant changes in parameters of diastolic function in females animals following estrogen deprivation or replacement" (338).

Participants and Methods: In this crossover study the researchers used echocardiography and Doppler techniques at baseline and during the washout periods to evaluate the effect of HRT (estradiol) on cardiac functioning. The subjects were 31 postmenopausal women (55–65 years) recruited by newspaper solicitation. The women used micronized estradiol (2 mg/d) for 12 weeks and were randomized to one of two treatment groups: fifteen women received estradiol in treatment period one and placebo in treatment period two; sixteen women were given placebos in treatment period one and estradiol in treatment period two. Women were excluded from the study if they had high blood pressure, heart disease, pulmonary disease, diabetes, thromboembolic disorders or elevated triglyceride levels.

▶ **Wakatsuki A, Ikenoue N, Izumiya C, Okatani Y, and Sagara Y.**

Effect of estrogen and simvastatin on low-density lipoprotein subclasses in hypercholesterolemic postmenopausal women. *Obstetrics and Gynecology*, September 1998; 92:367–372. **Type:** Experimental (clinical trial)

Focus: An investigation of the effects of estrogen and simvastatin on lipoproteins in postmenopausal women who have elevated cholesterol (hypercholesterolemia).

Conclusions: Women who received estrogen and simvastatin together had lower levels of LDL lipoproteins and triglycerides.

Findings:
• Combined therapy of estrogen and simvastatin was more effective at reducing lipoproteins than either estrogen or simvastatin alone.

- Combined therapy of estrogen and simvastatin reduced triglyceride levels.
- Estrogen therapy alone increased triglyceride levels.
- Women who received combined therapy of estrogen and simvastatin had reduced total cholesterol to target levels more than estrogen users.

Researchers' Comments: "Combined with estrogen, simvastatin reduced the estrogen-induced increase in total plasma triglyceride and might minimize the adverse effects of estrogen on LDL particle size" (371).

Participants and Methods: From April 1995 to March 1996, fifty-five postmenopausal Japanese women who had elevated cholesterol, participated in this three-month trial. The average age of the participants was fifty-five years. They were assigned randomly to one of three blinded treatment protocols: 0.625 mg/d conjugated equine estrogen; 5 mg/d of simvastatin, or 0.625 mg/d conjugated estrogen and 5 mg/d of Simvastatin. The women who participated in the study were assessed for general health, medical conditions, lifestyle, diet and medications. Cholesterol levels, triglyceride levels and lipoprotein levels were measured at baseline and at three months. Endometrial biopsies were also done at baseline and three months. Dietary counseling occurred before the study began. The women were to restrict fat consumption to less than 25 percent of daily total calories. Dietary changes did not, however, affect their cholesterol levels.

➤ **Walsh B, Schiff I, Rosner B, Greenberg L, Ravnikar V, and Sacks F.**

Effects of postmenopausal estrogen replacement of the concentrations and metabolism of plasma lipoproteins. *The New England Journal of Medicine,* October 1991; 325:1196–1204. **Type:** Experimental (clinical trial)

Focus: An investigation of the effects of HRT on the concentration and metabolisms of plasma lipids.

Conclusions: HRT (estrogen alone) lowers LDL cholesterol levels and increases HDL cholesterol levels. This may protect women receiving HRT from *atherosclerosis.* However, HRT increases triglyceride levels.

Findings:

- Triglyceride levels increased in women receiving HRT (conjugated estrogen, 0.625 mg/1.25 mg); this increase was dose dependent.
- Women receiving oral estradiol had a 30 percent increase in triglyceride levels.
- LDL cholesterol levels decreased from 15 percent in women who received conjugated estrogens.

- HRT (conjugated estrogen and oral estradiol) increased HDL levels, but transdermal estradiol did not.
- Oral estradiol (2 mg/d) lowered LDL cholesterol by 14 percent and increased HDL levels.

Researchers' Comments: "Estrogen therapy could exacerbate pre-existing *hypertriglyceridemia* and should be used with great care in patient with this disorder" (1201).

Participants and Methods: The research involved postmenopausal women (43–79 years) in two, randomized, double blind crossover trials with three treatment periods. In study one, 31 women participated and received a placebo and conjugated estrogens (0.625mg and 1.25 mg daily). These three treatments each lasted three months. Progestin (medroxyprogesterone acetate) was given for 10 days after the study to remove any abnormal endometrial growth. In study two, nine women received a placebo, oral micronized estradiol (2 mg/d), and transdermal estradiol (0.1 mg/biweekly). These three treatments each lasted six weeks. Progestin was given after each treatment to induce withdrawal bleeding. At baseline and at the end of each treatment period, the women were assessed for endogenous sex hormones (FSH, estrone, estradiol) total cholesterol, HDL cholesterol (three types), LDL cholesterol, very low density lipoproteins (VLDL) and triglyceride levels.

▶ **Walsh B, Kuller L, Wild R, Paul S, Farmer M, Lawrence J, Shah A, and Anderson P.**

Effects of raloxifene on serum and lipids and coagulation factors in healthy postmenopausal women. *Journal of the American Medical Association*, May 1998; 279:1445–1451. **Type:** Experimental (clinical trial)

Focus: An investigation of the effects of *raloxifene* and combined therapy on the risk of heart disease in postmenopausal women.

Conclusions: Raloxifene may reduce the risk of coronary artery disease by reducing LDL cholesterol without raising triglyceride levels. However, Raloxifene does not reduce the incidence of hot flashes.

Findings:
- Raloxifene, unlike combined therapy (estrogen + progestin) did not cause vaginal bleeding or breast tenderness.
- Raloxifene lowers LDL cholesterol, fibrinogen, and Lp(a) levels which are associated with an increased risk of heart disease.
- Raloxifene raised one kind of HDL cholesterol, but not both kinds that are increased by conventional combined therapy.

- Raloxifene reduced triglyceride levels; combined therapy raised triglyceride.
- Over half the women who received combined HRT (progestin + estrogen) experienced vaginal bleeding.

Researchers' Comments: "Almost half of HRT subjects experienced vaginal bleeding and approximately a third of HRT subjects experienced breast tenderness. Both of those symptoms caused many participants randomized to HRT to drop out of the study, and they also caused many women who have been prescribed HRT to stop taking it" (1451).

Participants and Methods: This six-month clinical trial (double-blind/placebo-controlled) involved 390 postmenopausal women (45 to 72 years) recruited through advertisements The study was conducted at eight sites in the United States. The women were assessed for general health, medical conditions and reproductive history. The women were randomized to one of four treatment protocols: (1) raloxifene hydrochloride, 60 mg/d (2) raloxifene hydrochloride, 120 mg/d (3) combined therapy, conjugated equine estrogen, 0.625 mg/d plus medroxyprogesterone, 2.5 mg/d (4) placebo. They were instructed not to change their diets. At baseline, 12 weeks and 24 weeks lipoproteins and coagulation factors were measured. The women were monitored thorough ten visits.

➤ **Waters D, Alderman E, Hsia J, Howard B, Cobb F, Rogers W, Ouyang P, Thompson P, Tardif J, Higginson L, Bittner V, Steffes M, Gordon D, Proschan M, Younes N, and Verter J.**

Effects of hormone replacement therapy and antioxidant vitamin supplements on coronary atherosclerosis in postmenopausal women. *Journal of the American Medical Association*, November 2002; 288:2432–2440. **Type:** Experimental (clinical trial)

Focus: An examination of the effects of HRT, vitamin C and vitamin E (alone or combinations) on the progression of coronary heart disease in postmenopausal women diagnosed with heart disease.

Conclusions: Postmenopausal women with diagnosed heart disease do not benefit from HRT, vitamin C or vitamin E either in combination or alone. Using these treatments may worsen a woman's coronary heart disease.

Findings:
- Women who received HRT and/or vitamin C and vitamin E had a decrease in the minimum *lumen* diameter of the vessels and subsequent reduced blood-flow through vessels compared with the placebo group.

- Women who received HRT had an increased incidence and risk of adverse cardiovascular events (e.g., heart attack, stroke, death).
- Mortality was lowest in the double placebo group (no HRT or vitamin C and vitamin E) and highest in the group receiving both HRT and vitamin C and vitamin E.
- Death, heart attack or stroke was diagnosed in 26 women in the HRT group compared with 15 in the HRT placebo group (**hazard ratio:** 1.90 for users/1.00 for nonusers).
- During the first year of follow-up, 5 or 6 deaths and 12 of the 18 death nonfatal heart attacks occurred in the HRT group.
- All-cause mortality was significantly higher in women who received antioxidant vitamins (vitamin C and vitamin E) than in the vitamin placebo group.

Researchers' Comments: "This trial fails to demonstrate that either HRT or antioxidant vitamin supplements provide cardiovascular benefit to postmenopausal women with coronary disease. In fact, potential harm was seen for both treatments" (2438).... Furthermore, these results strengthen the evidence that HRT causes cardiovascular harm during the first year or 2 of treatment" (2439).

Participants and Methods: This five-year trial, the Women's Angiographic Vitamin and Estrogen (WAVE) Trial, was a double blind and randomized study. The participants were 423 postmenopausal women (mean age of 65 years) with diagnosed coronary heart disease recruited between 1997 and 1999 at seven clinical sites in the United States and Canada. Exclusions from the study included the following: HRT within the previous three months, current use of vitamin C (more than 60mg/d), current use of vitamin E (30 IU/d), diagnosis of cancer, uncontrolled diabetes, a history of hypertension, planned or prior cardiac surgery, measured high triglycerides or high creatinine levels, a history of embolic conditions or stroke, and untreated osteoporosis. At baseline the women were assessed for general health, coronary artery status (angiographic data), blood chemistry, reproductive status, estrogen use and medications. At baseline and every twelve months, the participants were assessed for height, weight, blood pressure, waist circumference-to-hip ratio, pelvic examination, *Papanicolaou test*, mammography and physical exam. *Angiography* was performed at baseline and during follow-up to assess *stenosis*, lesions and structural changes in the vessels. The women were randomized to one of four treatment groups: (1) HRT placebo and vitamin placebo (2) HRT (conjugated equine estrogen 0.635 mg/d plus medroxyprogesterone acetate and/ or estrogen alone) and vitamin placebo (3) HRT placebo and vitamin C (500 mg/d) and vitamin E (400 IU/d) (4) HRT (conjugated equine estrogen

0.635 mg/d plus medroxyprogesterone acetate and/or estrogen alone) and vitamin C (500 mg/d) and vitamin E (400 IU/d). Follow-up phone contacts were made one month after randomization, and clinic visits were conducted at three months and six months intervals for the duration of the study.

> ## Writing Group for the Women's Health Initiative Investigators

Risks and benefits of estrogen plus progestin in healthy postmenopausal women (principal results from the Women's Health Initiative randomized controlled trial). *Journal of the American Medical Association*, July 2002; 288:321–333. **Type:** Experimental (clinical trial)

Focus: An investigation of the health benefits and risks of HRT (combined therapy).

Conclusions: The risks of using HRT (progestin + estrogen) exceeded the health benefits during a 5.2 year follow-up study in healthy postmenopausal women. Women who used HRT (combined therapy) had an increased risk of breast cancer, pulmonary embolisms, coronary heart disease and stroke; however, HRT lowered the risk of hip fracture and *colorectal cancer*. HRT should not be used for the prevention of treatment of coronary heart disease.

Findings:
- After 5.2 years of follow-up women who received HRT (combined therapy) had an increased risk of coronary heart disease (**hazards ratio**): 1.29 for users/1.00 for nonusers).
- After 5.2 years of follow-up women who received HRT (combined therapy) had an increased risk of breast cancer (**hazards ratio**): 1.26 for users/1.00 for nonusers).
- After 5.2 years of follow-up women who received HRT (combined therapy) had an increased risk of strokes (**hazards ratio:** 1.41 for users/1.00 for nonusers).
- After 5.2 years of follow-up women who received HRT (combined therapy) had an increased risk of pulmonary embolisms (**hazard ratio:** 2.13 for users/1.00 for nonusers).
- After 5.2 years of follow-up women who had received HRT (combined therapy) had a decreased risk of hip fracture (0.66 for users/1.00 for nonusers).
- After 5.2 years of follow-up women who received HRT (combined therapy) had a decreased risk of colorectal cancers (**hazard ratio:** 0.63 for users/1.00 for nonusers).

Researchers' Comments: " On the basis of these data the DSMB (Data and Safety Monitoring Board) concluded that the evidence for breast cancer harm, along with evidence for some increase in CHD (coronary heart disease), stroke, and PE (pulmonary embolism) outweighed the evidence of benefit for fractures and possible benefit of colon cancer.... Therefore, the DSMB recommended early stopping of the estrogen plus progestin component of the trial" (325).

Participants and Methods: Between 1993 and 1998, the Women's Health Initiative study recruited 161,809 postmenopausal women from 50 to 79 years to participate in a group of clinical trials: trials of low-fat diets, calcium and vitamin D supplementation, two trials of HRT (estrogen alone and combined therapy) and an observational study at 40 clinical centers in the United States. The estrogen plus progestin component was a randomized, blinded, primary prevention trial to assess the health benefits and risks of HRT (combined therapy). The participants were 16,608 postmenopausal women. The primary outcome for the trial of estrogen plus progestin was coronary heart disease, CHD death, and breast cancer; the secondary outcome was hip fracture. A global index summarized the balance of risks and benefits and included the two primary outcomes plus stroke, pulmonary embolism, endometrial cancer, colorectal cancer, hip fracture and death due to other causes. Women were excluded from the trial if they had any severe medical condition, prior breast cancer, other cancers within the last 10 years (except nonmelanoma skin cancer), low hematocrit or platelet counts, alcoholism or dementia. At baseline the women were assessed for general health, menopausal status, medical conditions, hormone use, blood chemistry. The women were randomly assigned to either receive a placebo, or conjugated equine estrogen (0.625 mg/d) and medroxyprogesterone acetate (2.5 mg/d). Participants were contacted six weeks after randomization to assess symptoms. Follow-up occurred every six months with annual clinic visits to assess health status including annual mammograms and breast exams. Electrocardiograms were collected at baseline and at follow-up years three and six. Formal monitoring of the study population began in 1997 with the expectation that the trial would last until 2005 with 8.5 years of follow-up.

▶ Wilson P, Garrison R, and Castelli W

Postmenopausal estrogen use, cigarette smoking and cardiovascular morbidity in women over 50 (The Framingham Study). *The New England Journal of Medicine*, October 1985; 313:1038–1043. **Type:** Observational (cohort)

Focus: An examination of the effect of HRT on morbidity from cardiovascular disease.

Conclusions: Women who used HRT had an increased risk of *cardiovascular morbidity* and *cerebrovascular* disease. Increased rates of heart attacks were found in women who used HRT and smoked. HRT use did not have a beneficial effect on mortality from all causes or cardiovascular health.

Findings:

- Women who received HRT (estrogen) had an increased risk of stroke (**relative risk:** 2.60 for users/1.00 for nonusers).
- Estrogen use was associated with total morbidity from cardiovascular disease (**relative risk:** 1.76 for users/1.00 for nonusers).
- The risk for coronary heart disease was higher in women who smoked and used HRT (**relative risk:** 4.17 for users who smoked/1.44 for users who did not smoke/1.00 for nonusers).
- Postmenopausal HRT for more than a few years elevated the incidence of vascular disease.
- Women who used HRT had an increased risk of cerebrovascular disease (**relative risk:** 2.27 for users/1.00 for nonusers).
- Women who used HRT had an increased risk of diseases of cardiovascular system.

Researchers' Comments: "Our findings suggest that the potential drawbacks to postmenopausal estrogen therapy should be considered carefully before recommending its widespread use" (1043).

Participants and Methods: The researchers reported information on a cohort of 1234 postmenopausal women, aged fifty to eighty-three years, who had participated in the Framingham Heart Study initiated in 1978. The data was obtained from the 12th biennial (every two years) examination between 1970 and 1972. Recorded estrogen usage (mostly conjugated estrogen) from biennial examination 8 through 12 was used to categorize the extent of estrogen exposure before eight years of observation for cardiovascular disease or death. For this report, the interval from examination 12 through examination 16 was the follow-up period (eight years). At the beginning of the study the women were assessed for general health, medical conditions, medications and estrogen use. HDL cholesterol, total cholesterol, LDL cholesterol, VLDL cholesterol, obesity, blood pressure, alcohol consumption, cigarette smoking and triglyceride level were also monitored. Follow-up involved a health assessment through reviews of clinical notes, hospital and physician records and death certificates on a biennial basis. A separate statistical analysis was completed for women who used HRT and smoked cigarettes. The dose of estrogen was not recorded uniformly during the exposure period, and therefore the potential dose effect was not examined.

> ### The Writing Group for the PEPI Trial.

Effects of estrogen or estrogen/progestin regimens on heart disease risk factor in postmenopausal women: the postmenopausal estrogen/progestin interventions (PEPI) trial. *The Journal of the American Medical Association*, January 1995; 273:199–208. **Type:** Experimental (clinical trial)

Focus: An examination of the effect of HRT on selected heart disease risk factors in healthy postmenopausal women.

Conclusions: Estrogen alone or combined therapy (estrogen + progestin) had a positive effect on lipoproteins and lowered fibrinogen levels without adversely affecting insulin or blood pressure. Unopposed estrogen was the best therapy for raising HDL levels. However, the association of estrogen (alone) therapy with endometrial cancer suggests that its use should be restricted to women who have had hysterectomies. Combined therapy is the approach recommended for women who have not had hysterectomies.

Findings:
- Women using unopposed estrogen had the highest increase in HDL levels, and women using estrogen + natural micronized progesterone had the best HDL levels in the combined therapy protocol.
- All forms of HRT produced higher levels of HDL cholesterol than the placebo; however, combined therapy did not have a substantial impact on long-term HDL levels. In all treatment groups HDL cholesterol decreased after the first six to twelve months.
- LDL Cholesterol levels decreased in all women who used HRT, but triglyceride levels increased in all HRT groups.
- Compared with the placebo group, total cholesterol levels were lower only in women who received conjugated equine estrogen plus medroxyprogesterone (combined therapy).
- Changes in fibrinogen levels varied between HRT users and the placebo group. However, the placebo group had the highest levels of fibrinogen.

Researchers' Comments: "Active treatment was not associated with an excess risk of breast cancer in PEPI women.... However, a 3-year trial is too short and the numbers of women in the PEPI trial are too small to exclude an excess risk with longer use" (207).

Participants and Methods: The PEPI trial was a three year, randomized and double-blind trial conducted at seven clinical centers in the

U.S. The participants were menopausal women, age 45 to 64 years. Women who had severe menopausal symptoms, used estrogen or progestin within three months of the trial, had thyroid disorders, cancer or heart diseases were excluded from the study. Between December 1989 and February 1991, the seven PEPI centers randomized 875 women who were assessed for social factors, medical history, medications, physical activity, cigarette and alcohol use and estrogen use. Treatment assignments were selected by computer, assigning each woman to one of five treatment groups: (1) conjugate equine estrogen (0.625mg/d) (2) conjugated equine estrogen (0.625 mg/d) plus medroxyprogesterone acetate (10mg/d for 1st 12 days) (3) conjugated equine estrogen (0.625mg/d) plus medroxyprogesterone (2.5mg/d) (4)conjugated equine estrogen (0.625mg/d) plus natural micronized progesterone (200mg/d for the first 12 days) (5) placebo. During follow-up the women were scheduled to be seen at three, six and twelve months the first year and thereafter every six months for a total of three years. Four endpoints were selected and measured in the women as indicative of heart disease risk: high-density lipoprotein cholesterol (HDL), systolic blood pressure, serum insulin and fibrinogen level.

3

Endometrial Cancer

Endometrial cancer is the abnormal growth and uncontrolled proliferation of the lining of the uterus. The lining has glands that respond to hormones. The endometrial lining is shed monthly during childbearing years. If proper shedding does not occur, a condition called hyperplasia may result with abnormal cell proliferation and the development of cysts. With even more stimulation without shedding, the endometrium can develop a precancerous condition called atypical hyperplasia. The symptoms of endometrial cancer include abnormal bleeding or postmenopausal bleeding. Endometrial biopsies are performed to diagnose the condition. Survival rates are high if detected early. Approximately 33,000 women are diagnosed with this cancer annually, and it occurs at a rate of about one in one-thousand postmenopausal women. It is the fourth most common cause of cancer in women in the United States. Sixty-eight years is the average age for endometrial cancer. Mortality rates have declined about 28 percent from 1973 to 1994. (http://www.nci.nih.gov)

Risk Factors and Endometrial Cancer

Risk factors associated with an increased risk of endometrial cancer include estrogen therapy or endogenous sources of estrogen unopposed by progesterone, obesity, infertility and irregular periods, and use of tamoxifen. HRT (estrogen alone) is associated with an increased risk of endometrial cancer and is now only prescribed to women who have had hysterectomies. Women who are overweight may be exposed to more endogenous estrogen because they have more fat cells, producing more estrogen; however some studies have not found that obesity is a risk factor and have found thin women at risk (Hulka et al., 1980). Infertility and irregular periods suggest that a woman is not ovulating and is probably exposed to too much estrogen and too little progesterone. During perimenopause when progesterone levels drop drastically, women are exposed to endogenous sources of unopposed estrogen and are therefore at more risk for endometrial conditions, such as hyperplasia. Although tamoxifen may help reduce the risk of breast cancer, it is associated with an increased risk of endometrial cancer. Paradoxically, it is an antiestrogen in breast tissue, but it stimulates the glands in the endometrium.

HRT and Endometrial Cancer

The relationship between unopposed estrogen and endometrial cancer is well established. Studies have consistently shown a strong association between the use of oral unopposed estrogen and the development of hyperplasia or endometrial cancer (Grady et al., 1995; PEPI Trial Writing Group, 1996). Most studies show that this risk increases with higher doses of estrogen and longer duration of therapy. Women who used HRT during the 1960s and 1970s experienced an increased incidence of endometrial conditions and cancer. Currently most women are given combined therapy (estrogen + progestin). Progestin, a synthetic progesterone, sheds the lining of the uterus avoiding hyperplasia and cancer. The long-term effects of progestin are not known because long-term studies on the effects of combined therapy have not been conducted. How much progestin or what regimen is the safest is still being debated. In one study, women who received progestin for ten days a month had an increased risk of hyperplasia and endometrial cancer (Beresford et al., 1997). However, another study reported no increase in hyperplasia with ten days of progestin a month (Paterson et al., 1980). More basic research is needed examining the effects of progestin on female biology.

Preventing Endometrial Cancer

Preventing endometrial cancer, like breast cancer, is not as clear-cut as preventing heart disease. However, there are a few measures that women can take. Exercising regularly, eating a healthy diet, having annual exams, undergoing biopsies or ultrasound for unexplained bleeding and limiting exposure to unopposed estrogen may reduce the risk of endometrial cancer. Oral contraceptives, breast-feeding and physical exercise have been associated with a lower risk of endometrial cancer. Oral contraceptives may prevent endometrial cancer by balancing the ratio of estrogen-to-progesterone. Breast cancer survivors who opt to use tamoxifen should be monitored for any endometrial changes. Postmenopausal women who choose to take HRT can avoid overexposure to estrogen by taking combined therapy. Treatments with progestin or natural progesterone have been used to treat hyperplasia. After menopause, growth promoting effects of estrogen on the endometrium are decreased because of lower estrogen levels. If a woman does develop the disease, a hysterectomy is usually done and depending on the state of the cancer, radiation and chemotherapy may also be used.

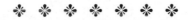

> **Antunes C, Strolley P, Rosenshein N, Davies J, Tonascia J, Brown C, Burnett L, Rutledge A, Pokempner M, and Garcia R.**

Endometrial cancer and estrogen use. *The New England Journal of Medicine*, January 1979; 300:9–13. **Type:** Observational (case-control)

Focus: An investigation of the relation between HRT and *endometrial cancer.*

Conclusions: HRT (unopposed conjugated estrogens) increases a woman's risk of endometrial cancer. Both conjugated estrogens and diethylstilbestrol were associated with an increased risk of endometrial cancer. Long-terms use (5 or more years) and higher doses (1 mg/d or more) were associated with endometrial cancer.

Findings:

- Women who received HRT (unopposed estrogen) had an increased risk of endometrial cancer (***relative risk estimate:*** 6.00 for users/1.00 for nonusers).
- Long-term users (5 years or more) had an elevated risk of endometrial cancer (***relative risk estimate:*** 15.0 for users/1.00 for nonusers).
- Increased risk of endometrial cancer was associated with both continuous and cyclic use of conjugated estrogens.
- A higher risk of endometrial cancer existed for all stages of the disease in women who received HRT (conjugated estrogens).
- Short-term (1 year of less) users of conjugated estrogen had an increased risk of endometrial cancer (***relative risk estimate:*** 2.20 for users/1.00 for nonusers).

Researchers' Comments: "We examine the question of whether or not swifter diagnosis of uterine cancer occurred among estrogen uses thus yielding a spurious association of the tumor with exogenous estrogen, but no such finding appeared in our series. Furthermore, the possible misclassification of estrogen-induced hyperplasia as cancer was not a problem in our series, and thus could not result in any important inflation of our risk estimates" (13).

Participants and Methods: The cases, 451 women, had been diagnosed with endometrial cancer and admitted to hospitals in the Baltimore area between January 1973 and February 1977. The information was obtained from hospital record, tumor registries, pathology records and discharge-diagnosis lists. Hospital interviews of cases and controls were performed. Endometrial cancer was validated by histologic reports from diagnostic or operative procedures. The cases were predominantly white women with an average age of 60.6 years. A control group of 888 women hospital patients were matched with the cases based on race, age, and date of hospital admission (with 6 months). One group of controls was drawn from hospital services other than obstetrics, gynecology or psychiatry. Another group of controls was obtained form gynecology services. All the participants were assessed for general health, estrogen use (duration, type, dosage), medicine use, medical history and lab results.

> **Beresford S, Weiss N, Voigt L, and McKnight B.**

Risk of endometrial cancer in relation to use of oestrogen combined with cyclic progestagen therapy in postmenopausal women. *Lancet*, February 1997; 349:458–461.

Type: Observational (case-control)

Focus: An assessment of the impact of HRT (oestrogen + cyclic progestagen) on the risk of endometrial cancer

Conclusions: Postmenopausal women who received combined therapy (estrogen + cyclic progestagen) had an increased risk of endometrial cancer when used for a long duration.

Findings:

• Women who received combined therapy had a higher risk of endometrial cancer than nonusers, even when progestagen was added for 10 or more days a month.

• Women, who received progestagen for 10 days or less a month as part of the HRT regimen, had an increased risk of endometrial cancer (*odds ratio:* 3.10 for users/1.00 for nonusers)

• Women who received progestagen for 10 to 21 days a month had a

slight increased risk of endometrial cancer (**odds ratio:** 1.30 for users/1.00 for nonusers)
- Long-term use of combined therapy (five or more years) with 10 or fewer days of progestagen was associated with an increased risk of endometrial cancer (**odds ratio:** 3.70 for users/1.00 for nonusers).
- The increased risk of endometrial cancer associated with combined therapy was not affected by the dose of estrogen.

Researchers' Comments: "Our results do not support the optimistic view of an overall lower risk of endometrial cancer being found with combined therapy than with no therapy" (461).

Participants and Methods: The cases were 832 women (45 to 74 years) in western Washington state who had been diagnosed with endometrial cancer as identified form a regional cancer registry (Cancer Surveillance System) from 1985 to 1991. The controls were 1526 women who were age and county matched with cases. The controls were identified by random digit dialing telephone calls within a tri-county area. Participants were assessed for medical conditions, general health, reproductive history, demographic characteristics and HRT (type, dosage, duration).

> **Clisham P, Cedars M, Greendale G, Fu Y, Gambone J, and Judd H.**

Long-term transdermal estradiol therapy: effects on endometrial histology and bleeding patterns. *Obstetrics and Gynecology,* February 1992; 79:196–201. **Type:** Experimental (clinical trial)

Focus: An examination of the long-term effects of transdermal estradiol on postmenopausal women.

Conclusions: Postmenopausal women who use transdermal estradiol plus medroxyprogesterone acetate have a lower incidence of hyperplasia than women who use transdermal estradiol alone.

Findings:
- Women who received transdermal estradiol (0.1 mg/d) alone had a higher rate of *hyperplasia* than women who received combined therapy (transdermal estradiol + progestin)
- Estradiol alone (18 percent hyperplasia at 1 year and 42 percent at 2 years); estradiol +10 mg of medroxyprogesterone acetate from day 13 to 25 of each cycle (4 percent hyperplasia at 1 year).
- Bleeding onset and duration were similar in both groups, and all subjects experienced bleeding during the treatment period.
- Most women averaged 5 days of bleeding per month.

Researchers' Comments: "E2 [estradiol] only therapy is safe, but the high incidence of hyperplasia formation (42 percent over 2 years) supports routine endometrial sampling" (201).

Participants and Methods: Women were recruited (newspaper advertisement) for this two-year clinical trial from the practices of physicians at the University of California at Los Angeles Medical Center. The subjects were assessed for medical history, general and gynecological health (estrogen use, menopause and endometrial status). Women were excluded from the study if they had abnormal Pap smears, endometrial biopsies, suspicious lesions or positive mammograms. The participants were randomized into one of two treatment groups. Group one received 0.1 mg of transdermal estradiol daily from 24.5 days of each month for a total of 96 weeks. Group two received the same dosage of transdermal estradiol plus 10 mg of medroxyprogesterone acetate (oral) from day 13 to 25 of each month. At baseline, vaginal bleeding and endometrial histology were described. Subjects kept records of bleeding history. Endometrial biopsies were done at 48 and 96 weeks. Of the sixty women who initially enrolled in the study, 46 women completed the trial. The study was not blinded.

➤ **Ettinger B, Bainton L, Upmalis D, Citron J, and VanGessel A.**

Comparison of endometrial growth produced by unopposed conjugated estrogens or by micronized estradiol in postmenopausal women. ***American Journal of Obstetrics and Gynecology***, January 1997; 176: 112–117. **Type:** Experimental (clinical trial)

Focus: An investigation of the effect of unopposed estrogen therapy on endometrial growth during long-cycle hormone replacement therapy.

Conclusions: Endometrial growth and unscheduled bleeding occurred in women who used full strength estrogens (micronized estradiol, 1.0 mg and conjugated estrogens, 0.625 mg) for HRT. Weaker estrogens (micronized estradiol, 0.5 mg) did not result in as much endometrial growth as full strength hormones. The growth of endometrial thickness in women receiving HRT varied widely.

Findings:
• Unscheduled vaginal bleeding was about half as likely to occur among women taking micronized estradiol (0.5 mg) as part of *long-cycle hormone replacement treatment.*
• Women who received conjugated estrogens (0.625 mg) had more unscheduled bleeding (28 percent) and scheduled bleeding (21 percent) than women who received micronized estradiol.

- Full strength estrogens (conjugated 0.635 mg and estradiol 1.0 mg) increased endometrial thickness more than weaker estrogens (micronized estradiol, 0.5 mg).
- Serum estrogen levels were not useful in predicting endometrial growth rates.
- 40 percent of the women using unopposed estrogen for as long as six months had endometrial thickness of 10 mm or more.

Researchers' Comments: "The considerable endometrial thickness that develops and the increased incidence of unscheduled vaginal bleeding that occurs should limit enthusiasms about widespread use of very-long cycle (24 week) treatment with full-strength estrogens" (117).

Participants and Methods: This six month trial involved 87 postmenopausal women (45 to 69 years) who were members of several Northern California Kaiser Permanente Medical Care Programs. The women were assessed for general health, medical conditions, reproductive history, medications, estrogen use and cigarette consumption. Women were excluded from the study if they had abnormal endometrial thickness, polyps or high triglyceride levels. The women were randomized to one of three treatment regimens: micronized estradiol (0.5 mg/d), micronized estradiol (1.0 mg/d) or conjugated estrogens (0.625 mg/d). Neither the participants nor the researchers were blinded to the treatment assignments. Estrogen treatment was given unopposed for 24 weeks and then medroxyprogesterone acetate was added for 14 days at a dosage of 10 mg daily. Endometrial thickness was assessed by vaginal probe ultrasonography at baseline and at 6, 12 and 24 weeks of treatment. For those women who were using HRT before the study, baseline measurements were done after medroxyprogesterone acetate (progestin) caused bleeding had stopped and prior to estrogen treatment. Endocrine tests for serum estrogens were performed at 6 and 24 weeks. Vaginal bleeding was measured daily on a scale of 0 to 4. Any bleeding that occurred during the unopposed estrogen phase was considered unscheduled bleeding and scheduled bleeding was any bleeding that occurred after the seventh day of progestin treatment.

> **Gelfand M and Ferenczy A.**

A prospective 1-year study of estrogen and progestin in postmenopausal women: effects on the endometrium. **Obstetrics and Gynecology**, September 1989; 74:398–401. **Type:** Experimental (clinical trial)

Focus: An investigation of the effects of estrogen and progestin on the endometrium in women receiving HRT.

Conclusions: Women who received combined therapy (estrogen +

progestin) had a lower incidence of hyperplasia than women who received estrogen alone.

Findings:

- Women who received conjugated equine estrogen alone (0.625–1.25 mg/d) for 25 out of 30 days had an increased incidence of hyperplasia (30 to 57 percent).
- Irregular, breakthrough bleeding occurred in 14 percent of the women who received combined therapy (conjugated equine estrogen, 0.625mg/d + progestin, 5 mg/d medroxyprogesterone).
- Women who received conjugated equine estrogen alone (1.25 mg/d) had an increased incidence of hyperplasia: 57 percent at the end of one year.
- Women who received combined therapy (conjugated estrogen + medroxyprogesterone) had menstrual like bleeding.
- Women who received combined therapy (estrogen + progestin) had an overall incidence of 4.4 percent for hyperplasia at 12 months despite the estrogen dosage.

Researchers' Comments: "This study has also shown that conjugated equine estrogen given without progestin is a very potent stimulator of the human endometrium" (401).

Participants and Methods: This one year, blinded study recruited participants from the Menopause Clinic of the Sir Mortimer B. Davis Jewish General Hospital and McGill University, Montreal, Canada. The women were assessed for general health, medical conditions and medications and reproductive history. All the women were postmenopausal and had pre-treatment endometrial biopsies. Of the 236 women who entered the study only 95 postmenopausal women finished the study. The women who dropped out of the study had various personal and medical reasons (excessive bleeding, nausea, bloating, headaches and leg cramps). The women were randomly divided into four treatment groups: (1) 25 women who received 0.625 mg/d conjugated equine estrogen and 5 mg/d medroxyprogesterone acetate (2) 27 women who received 0.625 mg/d conjugated equine estrogen and placebo (3) 20 women who received 1.25 mg/d conjugated equine estrogen 5 mg/d medroxyprogesterone acetate (4) women who received 1.25 mg/d conjugated equine estrogen and placebo. The women took the estrogen from days 1 to 25 of a 30-day cycle and the progestin or placebos were added to the regimen from days 15 to 25. The women recorded any vaginal bleeding and identified when the bleeding occurred. At six and twelve months the women were interviewed and endometrial biopsies were performed.

➤ **Grady D, Gebretsadik T, Kerlikowske K, Ernster V, and Petitti D.**

Hormone replacement therapy and endometrial cancer risk: a meta-analysis. **Obstetrics and Gynecology**, February 1995; 85:304–313. **Type:** Statistical (meta-analysis)

Focus: An assessment of the relationship of HRT to the risk of developing endometrial cancer or dying from the disease.

Conclusions: Women who received HRT (unopposed estrogen) for a duration of ten or more years have an elevated risk of endometrial cancer that persists even for five or more years after having stopped HRT. The risk of endometrial cancer varies with duration, dose and type of estrogen used. *Conjugated estrogen* carried a higher risk than *synthetic estrogens*.

Findings:

• Women who had used unopposed estrogen had an increased risk of endometrial cancer (***relative risk:*** 2.30 for users/1.00 for nonusers).
• Cohort studies showed a decrease in endometrial cancer; case-control studies showed an increased relative risk.
• Women who received unopposed conjugated estrogens had a greater risk of endometrial cancer than users of synthetic estrogens.
• The risk of death from endometrial cancer was elevated among women who used unopposed estrogen (***relative risk:*** 2.70 for users/1.00 for nonusers).
• Long-term users of unopposed estrogen had an elevated risk of endometrial cancer (***relative risk:*** 9.50 for users/1.00 for nonusers).

Researchers' Comments: "It has been suggested that endometrial cancer among estrogen users is not fatal, but the evidence concerning the risk of death from endometrial cancer among unopposed estrogen users has not been evaluated carefully" (304).

Participants and Methods: Thirty studies were selected from research published between 1970 and 1994. The researchers used MEDLINE, bibliographies and expert opinion. Studies were excluded from the analysis if "inappropriate" comparison groups were used, if risk estimates or *confidence intervals* were not available or if cases were few. When possible, the researchers abstracted information for risk estimates for duration, dose, type and regimen of HRT. The participants had used estrogen alone or combined therapy.

➤ **Gray L, Christopherson W, and Hoover R.**

Estrogens and endometrial carcinoma. **Obstetrics and Gynecology**, April 1977; 49:385–389. **Type:** Observational (case-control)

Focus: An investigation of the risk for endometrial cancer in women who receive HRT.

Conclusions: Women who used unopposed estrogen (all types) had an elevated risk of endometrial cancer. The risk was associated with longer use and higher dosages of estrogen.

Findings:

- Women who used estrogen for more than 10 years had an elevated risk of endometrial cancer (**relative risk estimate:** 11.5 for users/1.00 for nonusers).
- Women who used estrogen for less than five years had a slight risk of endometrial cancer (**relative risk estimate:** 1.20 for users/1.00 for nonusers).
- Women who received estrogens for five to nine years had an increased risk of endometrial cancer.
- Women who received conjugated estrogen dosages (1.25mg/d) had an elevated risk (**relative risk estimate:** 12.7 for users/1.00 for nonusers).
- Women who used conjugated estrogens had the highest risk of endometrial cancer (**relative risk estimate:** 3.10 for users/1.00 for nonusers).

Researchers' Comments: "The excess risk appears to apply to systemic estrogens of all kinds (intramuscular estrone, stilbestrol, ethinyl estradiol), not just conjugated estrogens. Second, there appears to be a positive dose-response relation between risk of the malignancy and both duration of use and strength of medication taken" (387).

Participants and Methods: The study group involved 410 women. The cases were 205 women who had been diagnosed with endometrial cancer and seen in one private practice from 1947 to 1976. These cases were matched with 205 controls according to age, parity, weight and year of surgery. The control group were women who had hysterectomies for benign condition during the same time that the cases had been diagnosed with endometrial cancer. The medical records of the subjects were assessed for information regarding estrogen use (type, dosage, duration), medications, general health, blood pressure, medical conditions, and reproductive history.

➤ **Hulka B, Fowler W, Kaufman D, Grimson R, Greenberg B, Hogue C, Berger G, and Pulliam C.**

Estrogen and endometrial cancer: Cases and two control groups from North Carolina. *American Journal of Obstetrics and Gynecology*, May 1980; 137:92–101. **Type:** Observational (case-control)

Focus: An investigation of the relationship between HRT and the risk of endometrial cancer.

Conclusions: Long-terms users of HRT (conjugated estrogens) had an increased risk of endometrial cancer. Non-obese, nonhypertensive women had the highest risk of endometrial cancer—five to eight times that of nonusers after 3.5 years of use.

Findings:

- Women who used HRT(conjugated or nonconjugated estrogen) for a short duration did not have an increased risk of endometrial cancer.

- Women who used HRT (conjugated estrogen) for a long duration (3.5 years or more) had an increased risk of endometrial cancer (***relative risk estimate:*** 4.20 for users/1.00 for nonusers).

- Obese, *hypertensive* women who used HRT did not have an increased risk of endometrial cancer compared with other normal weight women who received HRT.

- Estrogen use for 3.5 years or more increases the risk of endometrial cancer of early stage and low grade.

- The risk of endometrial cancer did not vary according to dosage or mode of administration (cyclic or continuous) of estrogen.

Researchers' Comments: "The lower risks for disease of advanced stage and grade with long-duration use of estrogen may be the result of closer medical surveillance and earlier diagnostic work-up"(101).

Participants and Methods: The cases in this study were 256 women who had been diagnosed with endometrial cancer from 1970 through 1976 and were receiving treatment at North Carolina Memorial Hospital. To match cases, two control groups were formed. A community control group involving 321 women and a gynecological control group of 224 women. The cases and controls were age matched within racial groups. The women were assessed for estrogen usage (type, dosage, duration), reproductive history and general health and medical conditions through patient interviews, hospital records and physicians' records.

➤ **Jelovsek F, Hammond C, Woodard B, Draffin R, Lee K, Creasman W, and Parker R.**

Risk of exogenous estrogen therapy and endometrial cancer. ***American Journal of Obstetrics and Gynecology***, May 1980; 137:85–90.

Type: Observational (case-control)

Focus: An investigation of the risk of endometrial cancer in women who receive HRT.

Conclusions: Women who used estrogen for five or more years had an increased risk for endometrial cancer.

Findings:

• The risk for endometrial cancer was higher in women who were white, nulliparous, hypertensive, diabetic, 60 years of age or more.

• The overall risk for all women in the study who received HRT (mostly conjugated estrogen) was 2.40.

• Women who received HRT and developed endometrial cancer had Stage 1, grade 1 lesions that were mostly treatable.

• Black women who used estrogen had a lower risk of endometrial cancer than white women who used estrogen (**odds ratio:** 0.60 for black women/2.90 for white women).

• Women who received HRT (mostly conjugated estrogen) for 5 to 10 years had the highest risk of endometrial cancer with a **odds ratio** of 4.80.

Researchers' Comments: "In the view of multiple studies which indicate an increased risk of endometrial cancer associated exogenous estrogen replacement therapy, it is difficult not to accept the existence of a definite relationship. The exact magnitude of the risk, however is much less clear and appears to vary according to the source of the control group, as well as the demographic and medical characteristics of these patients" (88).

Participants and Methods: The cases, 431 women diagnosed with endometrial cancer at Duke University Medical Center from 1940 to 1975, were women were identified through medical, pathological and physician records. Two control groups were formed from the files of the medical record's department. The first control group was 431 women who were matched with the cases by age, parity, race and area of residency. A second control group was formed and was matched with the cases based on the following criteria: age, parity, race, area of residency, weight, presence of diabetes and presence of hypertension. Cases and controls were assessed for estrogen use (type, duration), medications, reproductive history, medical conditions and general health.

▶ **Jick H, Watkins R, Hunter J, Dinan B, Madsen S, Rothman K, and Walker A.**

Replacement estrogens and endometrial cancer. *The New England Journal of Medicine*, February 1979; 300:218–222. **Type:** Observational (case-control)

Focus: An investigation of the incidence of endometrial cancer and its relationship to HRT.

Conclusions: Long-term HRT (estrogen) is associated with endometrial cancer.

Findings:

- The risk of endometrial cancer was much higher for current users of estrogen compared with nonusers.
- Among women with endometrial cancer, seven had taken progestin with estrogen.
- From 1975 to 1977 an abrupt downward trend in the incidence of endometrial occurred. This is associated with a reduction in HRT (mostly estrogen).
- Women who stopped estrogen therapy had a substantial drop in their risk of endometrial cancer within six months.
- Women who developed endometrial cancer had taken estrogens on a cyclic basis (with or without progesterone) at high dosages for at least five years.

Researchers' Comments: "The present study confirms that long-term replacement estrogen treatment is strongly associated with endometrial cancer" (220).

Participants and Methods: The subjects in this study were women (50 to 64 years) who were members of Group Health Cooperative, a large prepaid group practice in Seattle, Washington. The cases, 122 women diagnosed with endometrial cancer, were identified through the Cooperative's records from 1975 to 1975. The controls (122) were women who had been hospitalized for acute illness or elective surgery during time that the cases were diagnosed with endometrial cancer. The case and the controls were age-matched. All the participants were assessed for general health, medical conditions, medications, reproductive history, HRT (type, dose, duration). Although most of the women took estrogen alone, some did receive combined therapy (estrogen + progestin). Conjugated estrogen was used mostly; however, a few women used other estrogens (diethylstilbestrol, estradiol valerate and esterified estrogen). The dose range for conjugated estrogens was 0.3 mg/d to 2.5 mg/d.

➤ **Mack T, Pike M, Henderson B, Pfeffer R, Gerkins V, Arthur M, and Brown S.**

Estrogens and endometrial cancer in a retirement community. *The New England Journal of Medicine*, June 1976; 294:1262–1267. **Type:** Observational (case-control)

Focus: An investigation of the relation between HRT and endometrial cancer.

Conclusions: Women who use HRT (unopposed estrogen) are at an increased risk of endometrial cancer.

Findings:

- Conjugated estrogens were strongly associated with endometrial cancer.
- Women who used unopposed estrogen (0.625 mg/daily) had a higher risk of endometrial cancer than women who received lower dose, but risk ratios were greater than 3.00 even for low doses of estrogen.
- Women who had free interval days of no estrogen use had a lower relative risk of endometrial cancer than women who took estrogen continuously.
- Long-term users of unopposed estrogen (8 years or more) had an increased risk of endometrial cancer (*relative risk estimate:* 8.80 for users/1.00 for nonusers).
- Women who used unopposed estrogen (1 to 5 years) had an increased risk of endometrial cancer (*relative risk estimate:* 4.50 for users/ 1.00 for nonusers).

Researchers' Comments: "When estrogens are indicated, they should be given at the lowest effective dose for the shortest possible time" (1267).

Participants and Methods: The cases were 63 women who had been diagnosed with endometrial cancer and lived in a residential retirement community near Los Angeles. A survey was performed in the population in 1971 regarding health. Other sources of data included a cancer surveillance program in Los Angeles County, Los Angeles County death certificates. All participants in the study were assessed for drug use estrogen use (duration and type) and medical condition, through interviews, medical records and pharmaceutical records. Controls, 396 women, were selected from the same community as the cases. The cases and controls were matched according to age and martial status. Estrogen uses in this population were mainly conjugated estrogens (unopposed). They included diethylstilbesterol, ethinyl estradiol, estradiol, esterified estrogens, *cholortrianisene* and a few unidentifiable estrogen preparations.

▶ **McDonald T, Annegers J, O'Fallon W,
   Dockerty M, Malkasian G, and Kurland L.**

Exogenous estrogen and endometrial carcinoma: case-control and incidence study. *American Journal of Obstetrics and Gynecology*, March 1977; 127:572–579. **Type:** Observation (case-control)

Focus: An investigation of the relationship between estrogen use and the development of endometrial cancer.

Conclusions: Women who used HRT (conjugated estrogen) had an increased risk of endometrial cancer. The risk increased with larger doses (1.25mg/d).

Findings:

- Women who used conjugated estrogens for more than six months had an increased risk of endometrial cancer (*relative risk estimate:* 4.90 for users/1.00 for nonusers).
- Women who received conjugated estrogen (0.625 mg/d) for six or more months had an increased risk of endometrial cancer. This was found in users of conjugated estrogen (*relative risk estimate:* 1.40 for users/1.00 for nonusers).
- Women who received conjugated estrogen (1.25 to 2.5 mg/d) for six or more months had an increased risk of endometrial cancer (*relative risk estimate:* 7.20 for users/1.00 for nonusers).
- Obesity and nulliparity were associated with an increased risk of endometrial cancer in women who received HRT (estrogen).
- Women who used conjugated estrogen for more than three years had an elevated risk of endometrial cancer (*relative risk estimate:* 7.90 for users/1.00 for nonusers).

Researchers' Comment: "The incidence of endometrial carcinoma in Olmsted County does not show an increase over the three decades of this study. The lack of an increase could be explained by the relatively low use of long-term conjugated estrogen in this area" (579).

Participants and Methods: The participants in this study were recruited from medical records of the Rochester Project at the Mayo Clinic. The cases were 145 women in Olmsted County, Minnesota who had been diagnosed at with endometrial cancer since 1945. The 145 controls were age and residency matched with the cases and had been admitted to the medical facilities for general medical examinations. The cases and controls were assessed for general medical health, reproductive history, estrogen use (type, dosage, duration). The records on the participants were extensive with 86 percent of all the participants having as much as 20 years of medical care in the community.

➤ **Paterson M, Wade-Evans T, Sturdee D, Thom M, and Studd J.**

Endometrial disease after treatment with oestrogens and progestogens in the climacteric. *British Medical Journal*, March 1980; 280:822–824.
Type: Observational (cohort)
Focus: An investigation of endometrial cancer in women who had received combined therapy (oestrogen + progestogens).

Conclusions: Women who receive combined therapy (estrogen + progestin) have a lower incidence of hyperplasia than women who receive estrogen alone.

Finding:

- Women who received cyclical low-dose estrogen had a lower incidence of endometrial hyperplasia cancer than women who received cyclical high-dose estrogen.
- Women who received sequential combined therapy had a lower incidence of endometrial hyperplasia than women receiving estrogen alone.
- Women who received estrogen alone had a significantly higher incidence of all types of hyperplasia.
- Women who received combined therapy and took progestin for more than 10 days each month had no hyperplasia.
- The incidence of endometrial hyperplasia decreased with the longer a women received progestin during the month.

Researchers' Comments: "The length of treatment in our study was too short to allow any definite conclusion, but progestogens may reduce the risk of endometrial carcinoma" (824).

Participants and Methods: This twenty-one-month British study that was hospital based involved 745 women (average 50.2 years) who received different regimens of HRT for menopausal conditions. The women were assessed at baseline for general health, medical conditions, medications and estrogen use. They received an endometrial biopsy at baseline, six months and annually. Vaginal bleeding was defined as none, scheduled or unscheduled. Four treatment regimens were employed: cyclical low-dose estrogen for three weeks out of four, cyclical high-dose estrogen for three weeks out of four, sequential oral estrogen with progestin, continuous oral estrogen with progestin and subcutaneous estradiol implant.

➤ **Shapiro S, Kaufman D, Slone D, Rosenberg A, Miettinen O, Stolley P, Rosenshein N, Watring W, Leavitt T, and Knapp R.**

Recent and past use of conjugated estrogens in relation to adenocarcinoma of the endometrium. *The New England Journal of Medicine*, August 1980; 303:485–489. **Type:** Observational (case-control)

Focus: An investigation of the association between estrogen use and endometrial cancer.

Conclusions: The rate of endometrial cancer was increased in women who used conjugated estrogens (continuous or cyclical). The risk increased the longer the duration of use. Estrogen-free intervals did not lower the risk of endometrial cancer.

Findings:

- The risk of endometrial cancer did not increase with estrogen use of a year of less.
- Women who used HRT(conjugated estrogen) for five or more years had an increased risk of endometrial cancer (*relative risk estimate:* 6.00 for users/1.00 for nonusers).
- Women who took estrogen for one to four years had an increased risk of endometrial cancer (*relative risk estimate:* 2.60 for users/1.00 for nonusers).
- Women who had received HRT (conjugated estrogens) within a year and who had used estrogen for at least five years had an elevated risk of endometrial cancer (*relative risk estimate:* 8.80 for users/1.00 for nonusers).
- Long term estrogen users who had stopped use for two years still had an increased risk of endometrial cancer (*relative risk estimate:* 3.30 for users/1.00 for nonusers).

Researchers' Comments: "The present study shows that there is a residual effect of estrogen use on the risk of endometrial cancer long after such use has ceased. It is unlikely that this effect is due to chance, and it cannot be accounted for by selection bias due to uterine bleeding" (489).

Participants and Methods: The cases for this study were 174 postmenopausal women (50 to 69 years) who had been diagnosed with endometrial cancer between July 1976 and April 1979 in hospitals in the Eastern Seaboard, Kansas, California, Canada and Arizona. The controls, 453 postmenopausal women (50 to 69 years), had been admitted to the hospitals for the following conditions: orthopedic conditions, fractures, infections and other conditions. The cases and controls were similar in terms of race, religion, marital status and education. All the participants were assessed for medical history, reproductive history and estrogen use (type & dosages). Conjugated estrogens (Premarin) were the most commonly used estrogens. Women were excluded from the study if they had used HRT for a duration of less than three months or had used an unspecified female hormone.

➤ **Smith D, Prentice R, Thompson D, and Herrmann W.**

Association of exogenous estrogen and endometrial carcinoma. *The New England Journal of Medicine*, December 1975; 293:1164–1166. **Type:** Observational (case-control)

Focus: An investigation of the association between the incidence of endometrial cancer and the use of estrogen, and an examination of the risks associated with endometrial cancer.

Conclusions: HRT(estrogen) is associated with an increased risk of endometrial cancer.

Findings:

- Women who received estrogen had an elevated risk of endometrial cancer (*relative risk estimate:* 4.50 for users/1.00 for nonusers).
- The risk of endometrial cancer was lower in hypertensive and obese women than in women without these conditions.
- Women who developed endometrial cancer were not in a high risk group.
- Increased risk of endometrial cancer was associated with a longer duration of estrogen use and older age.

Researchers' Comments: "The present study provides a credible argument of the causative role of exogenous estrogen in the development of endometrial cancer" (1166).

Participants and Methods: The cases, 317 women (48 years or older), had been diagnosed with endometrial cancer from 1960–1972. The data was obtained from the Mason Clinic and Virginia Mason Hospital and the University of Washington Medical School Hospital, Seattle Washington. The cases were matched with equal number of controls according to age and year of diagnosis. The controls were women who had other gynecological conditions including ovarian cancer, cervical caner and vulva cancer. The participants were assessed for general health, medical conditions, medications and estrogen use (type, dosage, duration).

▶ **Weiss N, Szekely D, English D, and Schweid A.**

Endometrial cancer in relation to patterns of menopausal estrogen use. *Journal of the American Medical Association*, July 1979; 242: 261–264. **Type:** Observational (case-control)

Focus: An examination of endometrial cancer in relationship to estrogen use.

Conclusions: Long-term use of estrogens to reduce the risk of osteoporosis is associated with an increased risk of endometrial cancer.

Findings:

- Women who used estrogen for a long duration (11 to 14 years) had 20 times the risk of endometrial cancer compared with nonusers.
- Smaller dosages of estrogen (0.5mg/d or less) had a lower risk of endometrial cancer than higher dosages but still had an increased risk (*relative risk estimate:* 2.50 for users/1.00 for nonusers).

- Women who stopped taking estrogen had a decreased risk of endometrial cancer, but their risk was still higher than nonusers for up to ten years.
- Women who used estrogen in higher dosages had an elevated risk of endometrial cancer (**relative risk estimate:** 8.80 for users of 0.6 to 1.2 mg/d/1.00 for nonusers).
- An elevated risk of endometrial cancer occurred when estrogen was taken cyclically or continuously.

Researchers' Comments: "Lower dosages of estrogen are less hazardous than larger ones among long-term uses, but they produce a sizable excess risk nonetheless" (264).

Participants and Methods: Cases were 101 women (50 to 74 years) who had been diagnosed with endometrial cancer from January 1975 to April 1976 and were selected through the Cancer Surveillance System, a tumor registry serving Western Washington. The controls and cases, matched by race and age, were identified and interviewed through surveys distributed to female residents of King County, Washington. Cases and controls were assessed for general health, medical history, medications, reproductive history and HRT (type, dosage, duration). Conjugated and other estrogens were used most frequently.

> **Woodruff J and Pickar J (for the Menopause Study Group).**

Incidence of endometrial hyperplasia in postmenopausal women taking conjugated estrogens (Premarin) with medroxyprogesterone acetate or conjugated estrogens alone. *American Journal of Obstetrics and Gynecology*, May 1994; 170:1213–1223. **Type:** Experimental (clinical trial)

Focus: An investigation of the relation between the kind of HRT and the development of endometrial hyperplasia.

Conclusions: Women who received combined therapy (estrogen + medroxprogesterone acetate) had a lower incidence of *endometrial hyperplasia*.

Findings:
- No statistically significant differences existed between the lower-dose and higher-dose medroxyprogesterone acetate regimen or between the continuous combined or sequential treatments.
- Endometrial hyperplasia developed in 62 of the 1385 patient included in the evaluation at 12 months.
- The incidence of hyperplasia was lower in women who used combined

therapy (estrogen + medroxyprogesterone acetate) than in women who used estrogen alone.

• Five cases of endometrial hyperplasia were diagnosed in the two lower dose medroxyprogesterone groups.

• Two cases of endometrial cancer were found during the 13th cycle: one case had received combined therapy (higher dose, medroxyprogesterone acetate + estrogen); the other case received estrogen alone.

Researchers' Comments: "The results confirm the findings of previous studies showing that unopposed estrogen therapy increases the incidence of endometrial hyperplasia and that the addition of progestogen to estrogen replacement therapy significantly reduces the risk" (1217).

Participants and Methods: This study was a double-blind trial involving postmenopausal women (45–65 years) at nine sites in the United States and Europe. Approximately 1724 patents per group were participants in the trial. The women were randomly assigned to one of five treatment groups for one year. *Endometrial biopsies* were performed at baseline and during days 22 to 28 of cycle six and thirteen. Four different conjugated estrogens plus medroxy-progesterone acetate dosages were evaluated along with estrogen alone. The therapy was either cyclic or continuous therapy.

➤ Writing Group for the PEPI Trial

Effects of hormone replacement therapy on endometrial histology in postmenopausal women. *Journal of the American Medical Association*, February 1996; 275:370–375. **Type:** Experimental (clinical trial)

Focus: An investigation of the effects of HRT on the endometrium of postmenopausal women.

Conclusions: Estrogen therapy (0.625 mg/d) increased the incidence of hyperplasia. Combined therapy (estrogen + progestin) given cyclically or continuously protected the endometrium from hyperplasia.

Findings:

• Women who received estrogen alone were more likely to develop hyperplasia than women who received a placebo.

• Women who received combined therapy (conjugated equine estrogen + medroxyprogesterone acetate) or (conjugated equine estrogen + micronized progesterone) had similar rates of hyperplasia as those women given a placebo.

• Among the women who received estrogen alone (conjugated equine estrogen) 62 percent developed some type of endometrial hyperplasia during follow-up.

• Women who received estrogen alone had a higher incidence of all types of hyperplasia—simple, complex and atypical which are prognostic markers of the possible development of cancer.

• Forty-five women developed hyperplasia (complex and atypical) and estrogen alone therapy was stopped; seven hysterectomies were performed on women who had received estrogen alone (conjugated equine estrogen).

Researchers' Comments: "If the yearly occurrence of hyperplasia persisted in subsequent years, it would be anticipated that a majority of the women taking conjugated equine estrogen alone would have the more serious types of complex (adenomatous) or atypical hyperplasia after about five years of therapy. This finding raises serious questions about the safety of long-term conjugated equine estrogen only therapy in women with a uterus" (374).

Participants and Methods: This three year, multicenter, study involved 596 postmenopausal women ages 45 to 64 years. Women were excluded if they had a hysterectomy, breast cancer, endometrial cancer or any other cancer except nonmelanoma skin cancer. Participants stopped HRT two months before the first screening visit. The women were assessed for general health, medical conditions, reproductive history and medications. Endometrial biopsies were performed at baseline, at annual visits or unscheduled visits. The women underwent pelvic exams and PAPS tests during prestudy period. The groups were randomized to receive one of the following treatments in 28 day cycles: 0.625 mg/d conjugated equine estrogen, 0.625 mg/d conjugated equine estrogen plus 10 mg/d medroxyprogesterone acetate (for the first 12 days), 0.625 mg/d conjugated equine estrogen plus 2.5 mg/d medroxyprogesterone acetate (for the first 12 days) or 0.625 mg/d conjugated equine estrogen plus 200 mg/d micronized progesterone (for the first 12 days). During the study, the women were monitored for the development of hyperplasia. This study was initially a blinded investigation; however, protocol required unmasking for women with biopsy results classified as complex hyperplasia, atypical or cancer. Thirty-eight women were unmasked and of this group thirty one had received unopposed estrogen.

> **Ziel H and Finkle W.**

Increased risk of endometrial carcinoma among users of conjugated estrogens. *The New England Journal of Medicine*, December 1975; 293:1167–1170. **Type:** Observational (case-control)

Focus: An investigation of the relationship between endometrial cancer and the use of HRT (unopposed conjugated estrogen).

Conclusions: Women who use HRT (unopposed conjugated estrogen) have an increased risk of endometrial cancer.

Findings:

- The risk for endometrial cancer increased with duration of use of conjugated estrogens.
- Women who used unopposed conjugated estrogen for a short duration (1 to 5 years) had an elevated risk of endometrial cancer (**risk ratio estimate:** 5.60 for users/1.00 for non users).
- Women who received unopposed conjugated estrogens for a long duration (7 or more years) had an elevated risk of endometrial cancer (**risk ratio estimate:** 13.9 for users/1.00 for non users).
- Women who received unopposed conjugated estrogen for a moderate duration (5 to 7 years) had an increased risk of endometrial cancer (**risk ratio estimate:** 7.20 for users/1.00 for nonusers).
- Women who experienced a later menopause (age 51 years or more) had an increased risk of endometrial cancer.

Researchers' Comments: "Causal interpretation of the association between conjugated-estrogen use and the development of endometrial cancer has some biologic credibility." (1169).

Participants and Methods: The cases were 94 patients diagnosed with endometrial cancer at the Kaiser Permanente Medical Center in Los Angeles and reported to its tumor registry between July 1970 and December 1974. The controls were selected from the membership files of the Southern California Kaiser Foundation Health Plan population. Two control subjects were matches with the cases by age, residency and duration of the health plan membership. The most prevalent estrogen used by the women was unopposed conjugated estrogen; primarily, sodium estrone sulfate. The women were assessed for medical conditions, estrogen use, medications, general health and reproductive history.

➤ Ziel H and Finkle W.

Association of estrone with the development of endometrial carcinoma. *American Journal of Obstetrics and Gynecology*, April 1976; 124:735–739. **Type:** Observational (case-control)

Focus: An investigation of the relationship between HRT and the development of endometrial cancer.

Conclusions: Women who received HRT (conjugated estrogen) had an increased risk of endometrial cancer.

Findings:

- Women who received conjugated estrogens had an elevated risk of endometrial cancer (**risk ratio estimate:** 7.40 for users/1.00 for nonusers).

- Eighty-nine percent of the postmenopausal cases with endometrial cancer had used conjugated estrogens.
- Duration of estrogen use was associated with an increased risk of endometrial cancer.
- Long term use (3 or more years) of conjugated estrogens was associated with an elevated risk of endometrial cancer (**risk ratio estimate:** 9.20 for users/1.00 for nonusers).
- Women who used conjugated estrogens for a short duration (1 to 2.9 years) had an increased risk of endometrial cancer (**risk ratio estimate:** 4.60 for users/1.00 for nonusers).

Researchers' Comments: "It is important to note that the risk ratio was calculated for conjugated estrogens only, not for all estrogens. Since conjugated estrogens comprised the bulk of prescribed estrogen, adequate case numbers were available only for conjugated estrogens and not for other estrogen preparations" (736).

Participants and Methods: The cases, 94 women, were diagnosed with endometrial carcinoma from 1970 to 1974 at the Kaiser Permanent Medical Center in Los Angeles. For each case, two control subjects were randomly selected from a computer printout of the Health Plan subscribers in the geographic area served by the medical center. The cases and controls were age and residency matched. Women who had hysterectomies were excluded. All subjects are assessed for general health, medical conditions, reproductive history and estrogen usage (type, dosage, duration).

Osteoporosis

Osteoporosis is a disease of the bones involving demineralization, bone fractures and loss of stature. This occurs because bone resorption exceeds bone formation weakening the skeletal structure. The risk of osteoporosis increases in both aging men and postmenopausal women, particularly in those over 65 years. Of the 275,000 older people in the U.S. that have hip fractures every year, 20 percent die within a year from complications such as blood clots and infection (Rosen, 2003).

Osteoporosis in Women Is Affected by Many Variables

Osteoporosis, which involves an interplay of variables and causal factors, is a complicated condition that is not completely understood. Risk factors include existing fractures and low bone mineral density, increasing age, gender (women are at greater risk than men), race (Caucasians and Asian women are at higher risk), bone structure and body weight (small boned and lean women are at greater risk), menopausal and menstrual history (early menopause, cessation of menstruation due to anorexia, bulimia or excessive exercise), lifestyle (smoking, alcohol and tobacco consumption, lack of weight-bearing exercise, inadequate diet, low calcium and vitamin D intakes), medications and disease (corticosteroids, endocrine disorders, hyperthyroidism, rheumatoid arthritis, immobilization). The biomechanism of bone remodeling is complex and involves many factors. The body remodels old bone by breaking it down with cells called osteoclasts. Other bone cells called osteoblasts make new bone. With osteoporosis more bone destruction occurs than bone building. Osteoporosis is not a solely a disease of estrogen deficiency. A complex interplay and cascade of other enzymes, vitamins and signaling molecules are involved in bone destruction and formation, including parathyroid hormone, vitamin D, macrophage colony-stimulating factor, RANKL, osteoprotegerin and IFG-1 (Rosen, 2003). Malfunction of these biomolecules due to genetics or environment can set the stage for osteoporosis. Bone density levels and fracture risks vary between women and ethnic groups. In fact, Black women, despite age and estrogen status have a lower risk for osteoporosis. Thus, genetics and metabolism play an important role. In fact, genetic differences may account for up to 70 percent of the variability in human bone mass. Environment still plays a role—a woman's home can be a risk factor for fractures (e.g., unprotected staircases, throw rugs, icy entryways). Furthermore, poor balance and unstable movement can also increase a woman's risk of fracture. Ultimately, all women want to avoid falls despite bone density, since falling is the greatest risk for fractures.

HRT and Osteoporosis

HRT (estrogen alone) can slow bone loss in aging women. Future research will determine if HRT translates into fewer bone fractures and a better quality of life. The Woman's Health Initiative Study (Writing Group for the Women's Health Initiative Investigators, 2002) found that women who received combined therapy (estrogen + progestin) had a reduction in hip fractures. However, a lifetime use of HRT may be required to sustain its bone preserving benefit. If women stop taking HRT, the benefits on bone density cease after six years (Grady et al., 1992). The benefit of long-term use declines in women more than 75 years (Felson et al., 1993). The risks of estrogen (increased risk of breast cancer, cardiovascular problems, embolism, elevated triglycerides and gall bladder disease) may outweigh the benefits of treatment for osteoporosis especially when other treatments for osteoporosis are available without the risks associated with HRT.

Preventing Osteoporosis: DEXA, Pharmaceuticals, Diet, Supplements, and Exercise

A bone density test can aid a woman and her health care provider assess her risk of osteoporosis by measuring bone mass. DEXA (dual-energy,

X-ray absorptiometry) measures bone density of the hip and spine. This test can provide important data as a basis for treatment and prevention of osteoporosis for postmenopausal women.

Pharmaceutical drugs are available for the treatment and prevention of osteoporosis. Observational studies have found that HRT (estrogen) reduces the risk of hip and other types of fractures in women. Currently, the Women's Health Initiative is investigating fracture risk with long-term HRT. Because of the limited clinical trail data on the effects of HRT on fracture risk, HRT(estrogen or combined therapy) is not approved by the Food and Drug Administration (FDA) for the treatment of osteoporosis, only for the prevention of osteoporosis. Alendronate (Fosamax), risedronate, etidronate (Didronel), raloxifene, and calcitonin reduce fracture risk and have been approved by the (FDA) for the prevention and treatment of osteoporosis (Grady & Cummings, 2001). The downside of bisphosphonates (alendronated, risedronate, etidronate) is that some women experience stomach or esophagus problems. Raloxifene (Evista) increases bone density and reduces a woman's risk of breast cancer. However, like estrogen, it increases a woman's risk of blood clotting disorders. It can also exacerbate hot flashes. Calcitonin and bisphosphonates slow bone loss and are not associated with an increased risk of cancer. Some studies have also shown that statin drugs lower fracture risk; others have not found a reduction in fracture risk with statin treatment (van Staa T et al., 2001; Hennessy S et al., 2001). Experimental treatments using parathyroid hormone (Forteo) found that women receiving the hormone had substantial increases in bone mass up to 5 percent per year. Long-term studies and more trials are needed to assess the risks and benefits of treatment with parathyroid hormone and other osteoporosis treatments.

Diet, vitamins, minerals, and exercise affect a woman's risk of osteoporosis. An adequate diet and regular exercise can be part of a woman's lifestyle that guards against osteoporosis. Exercising moderately, doing weight-bearing exercise, eating a calcium-rich diet and maintaining a healthy weight can help protect women from developing osteoporosis. Supplemental minerals and vitamins may also help prevent osteoporosis: calcium-magnesium supplements, vitamin D, boron, zinc, copper, folic acid, and vitamin K. The Women's Health Initiative is investigating the effects of Vitamin D on osteoporosis. More research is also needed to assess the effect of supplements on osteoporosis.

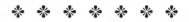

➤ Aloia J, Vaswani A, Yeh J, Ross P,
Flaster E, and Dilmanian F.

Calcium supplementation with and without hormone replacement therapy to prevent postmenopausal bone loss. *Annals of Internal Medicine,* January 1994; 120:97–102. **Type:** Experimental (clinical trial)

Focus: An evaluation of the effectiveness of calcium alone or calcium plus HRT in preventing early postmenopausal bone loss.

Conclusions: Calcium supplementation in a postmenopausal woman's diet retards bone loss from the neck of the femur but not in the spine. HRT(combined therapy) plus calcium is most effective at preventing bone loss.

Findings:
• Calcium supplementation was more effective than the placebo in preventing bone loss, but not as effective as HRT plus calcium.
• Bone mineral density of the spine and neck declined in the placebo group.
• Calcium supplementation in the diet retarded bone loss in women receiving HRT and those not receiving HRT.

Researchers' Comments: "Of the women on estrogen-progesterone-calcium, regular menses occurred in all but three patients. Three patients had mid-cycle bleeding, necessitating a *dilation and curettage* in one patient"(99).

Participants and Methods: This study involved 118 postmenopausal women. The women were assessed for general health, medical conditions, reproductive status, medications and estrogen use. Women were excluded if they had disorders known to affect bone metabolism or had been diagnosed with any malignancy. Each woman was randomly assigned to one of three treatment groups: HRT (conjugated equine estrogen, 0.625 mg/d for 25 days + medroxprogesterone, 10mg/ day 16 to 25), calcium carbonate or placebo. All women received 400 IU of vitamin D daily from a multivitamin. The initial daily calcium intake in the overall study group was 150 to 1263 mg/d and 222 to 806 mg/d in the calcium supplemented groups. Density of the spine, *radius* and *femur* were measured using photon absorptiometry.

➤ Cauley J, Lucas F, Kuller L, Browner W, and Vogt M.

Bone mineral density and risk of breast cancer in older women: the study of osteoporotic fractures. *Journal of the American Medical Association*, November 1996; 276:1401–1406. **Type:** Observational (cohort)

Focus: An investigation to determine if bone mineral density is associated with breast cancer.

Conclusions: Long-term exposure to estrogen in women as measured by BMD (bone mineral density) is an important risk factor for breast cancer. Furthermore, bone mineral density predicts the risk of breast cancer in older women. The researchers argue that the risk and benefits of HRT should be reevaluated especially in relation to BMD, *osteoporosis*, breast cancer and coronary heart disease.

Findings:

- High BMD is an indicator of estrogen exposure and is associated with breast cancer.
- The mean BMD was significantly higher among breast cancer cases than controls.
- Increased BMD was associated with an increased risk of breast cancer.
- Women with the highest BMD were at a 2.0 to 2.5 times increased risk of breast cancer compared with those with lower bone mineral density.
- Bone mineral density is an indicator of breast cancer risk in older women.

Researchers' Comments: "If women with normal BMD and normal or high *endogenous* estrogen were to take exogenous estrogen for other indications (e.g. to prevent cardiovascular disease), it is possible that the combination of high endogenous plus *exogenous* estrogens could increase the risk of breast cancer.... Our findings suggest that the risk of breast cancer associated with hormone replacement therapy may have been underestimated by previous investigators because osteoporosis is a primary indication for its use" (1407, 1408).

Participants and Methods: This study conducted from 1986 to 1988 involved 9704 women 65 years or older. Four medical centers in Baltimore, Minneapolis, Monongahela Valley, Pennsylvania and Portland, Oregon. participated in the study. The women were assessed for general health, medical conditions, medications, estrogen use, reproductive history and bone mineral density. A year after the baseline examination, the women were questioned about personal and family history of breast cancer. Follow-up information was obtained approximately three years later. During a second examination of the cohort (1988–1990), measurements of bone mass density of the femur and spine were made using X-ray absorptiometry.

➤ Christiansen C, Christensen M, and Transbøl I.

Bone mass in postmenopausal women after withdrawal of oestrogen/gestagen replacement therapy. **The Lancet**, February 1981; 1:459–461.
Type: Experimental (clinical trial)

Focus: An investigation of the effect on the bone density of the forearm when HRT is discontinued.

Conclusions: Annual bone loss after discontinuation of HRT (estrogen + progestin) was the same as women who had never received HRT. Temporary use of HRT after menopause will have a beneficial affect on bone mass.

Findings:
- Bone mineral density increased by 3.7 percent for three years in women receiving HRT (estrogen + progestin).
- Bone mineral density decreased in women who received a placebo by 5.7 percent during a three year period.
- Bone mass in women who received HRT was 8 percent higher than in the placebo group after therapy for three years.
- HRT resulted in increased bone mineral density of 1.9 percent after one year of treatment.
- Withdrawal of HRT resulted in an annual decrease in bone mineral density of 2.3 percent.

Researchers' Comments: "The acceleration of bone loss after withdrawal of female hormones reported by Lindsay et al. and by Horsman et al. does not accord with our results" (461).

Participants and Methods: This Danish trial involved 114 postmenopausal who had undergone menopause within six months to three years. The women were selected by questionnaire and medical screening. The women were assessed for general health, medical conditions, serum estradiol levels and reproductive status. Bone mineral density of the forearm was determined at baseline and at every three months for three years using photon absorptiometry. In the first study group the women were randomized into one of three groups: HRT (estradiol 4 mg for days 1–12 and *estriol* 2 mg days 13–22), HRT (estradiol 4 mg; and estriol 0.5 mg) or placebo. After two years of treatment, the women were asked to continue in a second study for one year. During both studies the women received 500 mg of calcium per day. Of the 114 women, 94 completed the first two years of the study and 94 participated in the second part of the study with 77 women completing it.

▶ **Cummings S, Browner W, Bauer D, Stone K, Ensrud K, Jamal S, and Ettinger B (for the Study of Osteoporotic Fractures Research Group).**

Endogenous hormones and the risk of hip and vertebral fractures among older women. *The New England Journal of Medicine*, September 1998; 339:733–738. **Type:** Observational (cohort)

Focus: A comparison of the endogenous estrogen levels in women (65 years or more) who had fractures with a control group of women from the same

Conclusions: Postmenopausal women with an undetectable level of *serum estradiol* (< 5 pg per milliliter/18 pmol per liter) have an increased risk of hip or vertebral fractures cohort. Maintaining low, but detectable estrogen levels in the blood may reduce the risk of fracture without increasing the risk of breast or endometrial cancer.

Findings:

- Higher endogenous levels of *estrone* was associated with an increased risk of vertebral fractures.
- Women who had low serum vitamin D concentrations had an increased risk of hip but not vertebral fractures.
- Women who had serum total estradiol concentrations of less than 5 pg milliliters have an increased risk of hip and vertebral fractures. This result was independent of bone density.
- Higher serum concentration of *globulin* (1.0 µg per deciliter/34.7 nmol per liter) was associated with a greater risk of fractures: hip fractures **(relative risk:** 2.00) and vertebral fracture **(relative risk:** 2.30). This result was independent of bone density.
- Women who had undetectable serum estradiol concentrations and globulin serum levels of more than 1 µg per deciliter, had an increased risk of hip fractures **(relative risk:** 6.90) and an increased risk of vertebral fractures **(relative risk:** 7.90).

Researchers' Comments: "Our results are consistent with the view that vertebral and hip fractures are manifestations of estradiol deficiency in older, as well as younger postmenopausal women" (737).

Participants and Methods: The women (9704) were from the Study of Osteoporotic Fractures, whose cohort was recruited from population-based listing in Baltimore, Minneapolis, Pittsburgh and Portland. This study conducted from 1986 to 1988 involved 133 postmenopausal women (65 years or older) who had hip fractures, 138 postmenopausal women who had vertebral fractures, and 359 women who were the control group. Black women, women receiving HRT, women who had undergone hip replacement, or women unable to walk were excluded from the study. All the participants were assessed for general health, medical conditions, medications, estrogen and vitamin use, dietary intake of calcium and tobacco use. X-ray films of the thoracic and lumbar spine were obtained, and bone mineral density of the heel was measured using single-photon absorptionmetry. Blood tests were performed to measure serum estradiol levels, globulin, estrone, testosterone, parathyroid hormone and vitamin

D levels. The study group was older, weighed less and had lower bone density at base line than the control group; however, the data was adjusted for age and weight.

➤ Ettinger B, Genant H, and Cann C.

Long-term estrogen replacement therapy prevents bone loss and fractures. *Annals of Internal Medicine*, March 1985; 102:319–324. **Type:** Observational (case-control)

Focus: An investigation of the effect of estrogen replacement therapy in preventing postmenopausal bone loss and bone fractures.

Conclusions: Long-term estrogen replacement offers protection against bone loss and fracture.

Findings:

• Women who received HRT had greater bone mineral density than nonusers: 54.2 percent greater spinal bone mineral density and 19.4 percent greater *metacarpal cortical* thickness.
• The total number of fractures was 53.7 percent lower in women receiving estrogen.
• Wrist fractures were less common in estrogen users; however, only vertebral fractures were statistically significant.
• Hip fractures (0.8 percent) were observed in hormone users and nonusers.
• Vertebral crush fractures were detected in 2.5 percent of the estrogen users and 6.6 percent of the nonusers.

Researchers' Comments: "Estrogen therapy may not confer the same degree of protection in all parts of the skeleton.... [W]e saw the greatest reductions in spinal compression fracture prevalence and spinal fracture index, but only a small decrease in wrist fractures" (323).

Participants and Methods: The data for this study were obtained using computerized pharmacy records at a San Francisco Medical Center for the years 1968 to 1971. The cases were 242 women receiving HRT (estrogen and combined therapy) and 242 matched control who did not use HRT. The average age of the participants was 73 years. The women were followed until 1985 to determine the incidence of fractures. They were assessed for demographic data, general health, medical conditions, reproductive history, estrogen use, medications and cigarette consumption. The women whose records showed regular estrogen use up to the time of the study, were contacted and asked to have bone mineral density tests using *photon absorptiometry* and *quantitative computed tomography*. The women using estrogen were more likely to be nulliparous and 1.5 years older at the time of menopause and at the end of follow-up. Estrogens used included conjugated equine estrogen and ethinyl estradiol. Combined therapy (progestin + estrogen) was used by 5.8 percent of the HRT users: 16.6 percent of the women used 0.3 to 0.624 mg/d, 68.1 percent of the women used more than 1.25 mg/d.

➤ Ettinger B, Genant H, and Cann C.

Postmenopausal bone loss is prevented by treatment with low-dosage estrogen with calcium. *Annals of Internal Medicine,* January 1987; 106:40–45. **Type:** Observational (cohort)

Focus: An assessment of the protective effects of calcium supplements given alone or in combination with estrogen on three skeletal sites.

Conclusions: Women who receive estrogen plus calcium supplements have a slight increase in bone density. Calcium supplements alone do not protect against bone loss that occurs at menopause.

Findings:
• Women who did not receive estrogen therapy had a decrease in bone density.
• Women who received HRT, conjugated estrogen (0.3 mg/d) with calcium supplements (1500 mg/d) had a slight increase in bone mass (2.3 percent).
• No significant change in bone density was measured in women receiving estrogen plus calcium.
• Women who had their ovaries surgically removed had higher bone loss than women who had a normal menopause.
• Age, years postmenopausal, race, height, weight, parity, smoking, calcium intake and physical activity were not significantly related to loss of bone density in the spine.

Researchers' Comments: "Our present study ... refutes the claim that a high-calcium diet will prevent the rapid bone loss that occurs in early menopause.... We recommend that women receiving estrogen replacement therapy be given the smallest effective dosage, because the incidence of side effects is dose related" (45).

Participants and Methods: The participants (Caucasian, Asian and Hispanic) were recruited from the Kaiser Permanente Health Plan in San Francisco, California for this two-year study. Seventy-three postmenopausal women formed the final cohort. The participants were assessed for general health, cigarette and alcohol consumption, physical activity, medications, medical conditions, estrogen use and reproductive status. Women were excluded if they had bone disease or a medical condition contributing to bone disease. Each woman was allowed to select her therapy: conjugated estrogen (0.3 mg/d) plus oyster shell calcium (1500 mg/d), conjugated estrogen (0.3 mg/d) plus progestin (10 mg medroxyprogesterone or 5 mg norethindrone acetate) plus oyster shell calcium (1500 mg/d), oyster shell calcium alone (1500 mg/d) and no therapy. Estrogen was given for 25 days of each month, and for most women a progestogen was added from day 16 through day 25. Eight women were given 0.625 mg/d conjugated estrogen because they had low bone mineral density in their spines at baseline. Bone mineral density was measured at three skeletal sites (spine, wrist, forearm) using single-photon absorptiometry at baseline, year one and at the end of the treatment period.

▶ **Ettinger B, Black D, Mitlak B, Knickerbocker R, Nickelsen T, Genant H, Christiansen C, Delmas P, Zanchetta J, Stakkestad J, Glüer C, Krueger K, Cohen F, Eckert S, Ensrud K, Avioli L, Lips P, and Cummings S (for the Multiple Outcomes of Raloxifene Evaluation [MORE] Investigators).**

Reduction of vertebral fracture risk in postmenopausal women with osteoporosis treated with raloxifene, results from a 3-year randomized clinical trial. *Journal of the American Medical Association*, August 1999; 282:637–645. **Type:** Experimental (clinical trial)

Focus: An evaluation of the effect of HRT (raloxifene) on the risk of vertebral and nonvertebral fractures.

Conclusions: After three years of treatment, postmenopausal women with osteoporosis have an increase in bone mineral density in the spine and in the hip. Raloxifene appears to reduce the risk of vertebral fractures and reduces bone turnover.

Findings:
- Of the participants, 7.4 percent had at least one new vertebral fracture: 10.1 percent of the placebo group, 6.6 percent of the 60 mg/daily raloxifene group, and 5.4 percent of the 120 mg/daily raloxifene.
- Risk reduction of vertebral fractures was found in both raloxifene groups (*relative risk:* 0.7 for 60 mg raloxifene/0.5 for 120 mg raloxifene/1.00 for nonusers).
- Women who received raloxifene had an increased risk of venous thromboembolism (*relative risk:* 3.10 for users/1.00 for placebo group).
- Bone mineral density increased after 36 months in the women who received raloxifene: 2.1 percent and 2.6 percent at the *femoral neck* and

spine in the 60 mg raloxifene group/2.4 percent and 2.7 percent at the femoral neck and spine in the 120 mg raloxifene group.

- Women who received raloxifene had a lower incidence of breast cancer (*relative risk:* 0.30 for both raloxifene groups/ 1.00 for placebo group.
- No reduction of nonspine fractures was observed during the three-year trial.

Researchers' Comments: "Our study supports previous observations that the effect of fracture reduction is not clearly related to increase in bone mineral density, suggesting that other factors also contribute to prevention of fractures. Indeed, lower bone turnover in elderly women is associated with decreased risk of hip fractures independent of bone density" (643).

Participants and Methods: This three-year trial recruited 7705 postmenopausal women (31–81 years) with osteoporosis. The women were enrolled at 180 centers in twenty-five countries. Of the participants, 95.7 percent were Caucasian. The women were assessed for general health, medical history and medications and blood chemistry. All the women received calcium and cholecalciferol supplements, which might have affected the risk of fractures in both placebo and raloxifene groups. Bone mineral density, using *dual-energy* X-ray *absorptiometry (DEXA)* was performed at baseline and annually. Vertebral and fractures were assessed using radiography at baseline, 24 months and 36 months. Mammographies were performed at baseline, at one year (optional) and year two and three. The women were randomized into two study groups. Study group one included women with hip and spine bone mineral density *t* score below −2.5. The women in the second study group had low bone mineral density and had experienced one or more mild to severe vertebral fractures. Women were excluded for the following conditions: bone disease other than osteoporosis, severe postmenopausal symptoms or abnormal bleeding, endometrial, breast or skin cancer, a history of thromboembolism, estrogen use within the previous two months, androgen use or medication for osteoporosis within the past six months, abnormal liver tests or consumption of more than four alcoholic drinks per day. Within each study group, women were randomly assigned to receive a placebo, 60 mg/d raloxifene or 120 mg/d raloxifene. All the participants received 500 mg of calcium daily and 400 to 600 IU of cholecalciferol (vitamin D-3).

► **Felson D, Zhang Y, Hannan M, Kiel D, Wilson P, and Anderson J.**

The effects of postmenopausal estrogen therapy of bone density in elderly women. *The New England Journal of Medicine*, October 1993; 329:1141–1146. **Type:** Observational (cross-sectional)

Focus: An examination of elderly women to determine whether or not postmenopausal estrogen therapy affected bone density.

Conclusions: If women want to preserve bone density, they need to take estrogen for at least seven years after menopause. Women, 75 years or older, the age group most at risk for fracture, may receive little or no benefit from therapy of this duration. The long-term effect of postmenopausal estrogen therapy on bone density is not known.

Findings:

- Estrogen therapy begun soon after menopause decreases or reverses bone loss characteristic of those years.
- Smoking has a negative impact on the benefits of long-term estrogen therapy.
- The density of the shaft of the radius and the ultra distal radius was greater with increasing duration of estrogen therapy. This was especially noticeable in women who had taken estrogen for at least 10 years.
- Among the women who received HRT for a period of 3–4 years, average bone density was no different from women who had not received HRT.
- Nonsmokers who had taken HRT showed higher bone density at all sites.

Researchers' Comments: "Although five years of estrogen therapy has been suggested, on the basis of epidemiologic studies of estrogen therapy and hip fracture in which women who had taken estrogen for different periods of time who were grouped together, there are insufficient data to support this recommendation" (1141).

Participants and Methods: In 1948 the Framingham Study began with the goal of evaluating risk factors for heart disease. It involved 1164 surviving Caucasian subjects (488 men and 716 women). The participants had been examined every two years and by 1988 half of the original cohort had died. The Framingham Osteoporosis Study was a part of the biennial examination performed in 1988 and 1989. The women, 68 to 96 years, were assessed for medical conditions, general health, reproductive history, estrogen use, age, weight, height, smoking, physical activity and bone mineral density. The researchers excluded women from analysis who had a history of fractures or osteoporosis prior to estrogen therapy. The women were followed prospectively.

➤ **Gallagher J, Goldgar D, and Kable W.**

Effect of progestin therapy on cortical and trabecular bone: comparison with estrogen. *The American Journal of Medicine*, February 1991; 90:171–177. **Type:** Experimental (clinical trial)

Focus: An investigation of the effect of progestin on bone mineral density in postmenopausal women who receive HRT.

Conclusions: Progestin reduces the rate of bone loss in *cortical* areas of the skeleton. However, it does not reduce bone loss in the *trabecular* area of the spine. Estrogen therapy is the most effective treatment in slowing bone loss in postmenopausal women. It reduces the rate of bone loss in cortical and trabecular bone.

Findings:

- Women who received the placebo lost bone at all sites.
- Women who received progestin (Provera) had no change in total body calcium but had a decrease in radial density of the cortical bones in the hand and the trabecular bone of the spine.
- Combined therapy (estrogen + progestin) worked as well as estrogen (Premarin) alone in its effect on bone. Estrogen therapy alone increased spine density and total body density but not *radius* density.
- Estrogen (alone) therapy and combined therapy decreased serum cholesterol levels.
- Estrogen (alone) therapy increased triglyceride levels; progestin (alone) therapy decreased triglyceride levels, but combined therapy did not change triglyceride levels.

Researchers' Comments: "The combination of half the dose of Premarin (0.3mg) and half the dose of Provera (10 mg) was almost equally effective as the 0.6 mg dose of estrogens in preventing bone loss from the spine" (176).

Participants and Methods: This two-year, clinical trial involved 81 postmenopausal women (46 to 56 years) solicited from advertisements at local businesses and newspapers. The women were assessed for general health, diet, medical conditions (including any conditions or drugs that would affect calcium metabolism), estrogen use, medications and reproductive history. About half the subjects in each group previously had hysterectomies. Blood tests and general biochemical screens were performed in all the women. The women were randomized into one of four treatment groups: conjugated estrogens (Premarin, 0.6 mg/daily), medroxyprogesterone (Provera, 20 mg/d), conjugated estrogens (Premarin, 0.3 mg/d + Provera 10 mg/d) or placebo. The Provera and placebo groups had identical matching pills so that those two treatment groups were double-blind. The Premarin and combined therapy groups were single-blind because the pills did not look the same. All medications were given for 23 days on and five days off in a 28-day cycle. The women were also given supplemental calcium carbonate (600 mg/d). Evaluations were performed at six-months intervals which included physical exams and bone density measurements (using single and dual-photon absorptiometry and metacarpal radiogrammetry). At baseline and at two years, 60 of the subjects underwent CAT scans.

> ➤ **Genant H, Baylink D, Gallagher J,
> Harris S, Steiger P, and Herber M.**

Effect of estrone sulfate on postmenopausal bone loss. *Obstetrics and Gynecology*, October 1990; 76:579–584. **Type:** Experimental (clinical trial)

Focus: An evaluation of the dose-response relationship between *estrone sulfate* and the prevention of bone loss in postmenopausal women.

Conclusions: Estrone sulfate (0.625 mg/d) plus Calcium (1000 mg/d) was the minimum dosage effective at preventing bone loss in the spine.

Findings:
- After one year of treatment bone mineral density increased by 1.9 percent in women receiving HRT (estrone sulfate, 0.625 mg/d). Women who received the placebo loss bone at the rate of 0.9 percent annually.
- Women who received HRT (estrone sulfate, 0.3 mg/d) were similar to the placebo group in loss of bone mineral density.
- HRT (estrone sulfate, 0.625mg or 1.25 mg) reduced total cholesterol and LDL cholesterol and increased HDL cholesterol.
- Hyperplastic endometrial changes were seen in two women: one receiving estrone sulfate (1.25 mg/d) and the other receiving estrone sulfate (1.25 mg/d).

Researchers' Comments: "Estrogen use by a postmenopausal woman stabilizes bone density by preventing further loss. In fact, when estrogens are given to a woman experiencing rapid bone loss, a small increment in bone mass is often seen" (583).

Participants and Methods: This two-year trial (double blind) involved 122 women who had undergone an oophorectomy within six months to four years of the study's initiation and participated in the bone mineral density analyses. The participants were assessed for general health, estrogen use, medical conditions, reproductive status and medications. Women were excluded for the following condition: high blood pressure, obesity and other disease or conditions that might influence calcium metabolism. The women were given an endometrial biopsy at baseline and at one year. Physical examinations were done at the first visit and at three-month intervals and laboratory tests were done annually. Bone mineral density measurements of the spine were taken at baseline, six months and twelve months using quantitative computed tomography. Participants were randomized to receive one of the following treatments: estrone sulfate (0.3 mg/d), estrone sulfate (0.625 mg/d) or placebo. Estrone sulfate was taken cyclically with one tablet nightly for days 1–25 and six days of no therapy. All the participants received 1000 mg of calcium/daily.

➤ **Grey A, Stapleton J, Evans M, Tatnell M, and Reid I.**

Effect of hormone replacement therapy on bone mineral density in postmenopausal women with mild primary hyperparathyroidism. *Annals of Internal Medicine*, September 1996; 125:360–367. **Type:** Experimental (clinical trial)

Focus: An examination the effects of estrogen-progestin therapy (HRT) on bone mineral density and biochemical measurements in postmenopausal women diagnosed with primary hyperparathyroidism.

Conclusions: HRT reduced urinary calcium excretion to a normal level. The researchers also found that HRT increased bone mineral density and bone turnover in postmenopausal women with mild primary *hyperparathyroidism*.

Findings:
- HRT increased bone mineral density throughout the skeleton in postmenopausal women with mild hyperparathyroidism.
- Combined therapy (estrogen + progestin) reduces the risk of fractures in women with primary hyperthyroidism.
- Markers of bone turnover decreased in the HRT group.
- Urinary markers of bone reabsorption decreased in the women using HRT.
- Vaginal bleeding and *mastalgia* occurred more often in women receiving HRT.

Researchers' Comments: "Our findings suggest that hormone replacement therapy should be considered an alternative to parathyroidectomy...." (376)

Participants and Methods: Thirty-three postmenopausal women with mild, primary hyperparathyroidism participated in and completed this clinical trial initiated from the Auckland Hospital's Endocrinology clinic in Auckland, New Zealand. Seventeen women received HRT and sixteen women received a placebo. Hypercalcemia was detected through blood tests. The women were randomly assigned to receive either conjugated estrogen (0.625mg/d) plus medroxyprogesterone (5mg/d) or a placebo. The data included bone mineral densities of the entire body, and biochemical indicators of bone turnover and calcium baselines. Measurements were taken every six months using X-ray absorptiometry. The biochemical measurements were recorded at baseline, six months and two years.

➤ **Harris S, Genant H, Baylink D, Gallagher C, Karp S, McConnell M, Green E, and Stroll R.**

The effects of estrone (Ogen) on spinal bone density of postmenopausal women. *Archives of Internal Medicine*, October 1991; 151:1980–1984. **Type:** Experimental (clinical trial)

Focus: An investigation of the effects of cyclical treatment with estrogen (estrone sulfate) plus calcium carbonate on spine bone density.

Conclusions: Estrogen (estrone sulfate) was effective at preventing bone loss at dosages of 0.625 mg/d and 1.25 mg/d when supplemented with calcium. However, the 1.25 mg/d (estrone sulfate) group did have some bone loss at 24 months. The 0.3 mg/d treatments were not effective at preventing bone loss.

Findings:
* Women who received HRT (estrone sulfate/1.25 mg/d) had no significant spine bone loss at 24 months.
* Women who received HRT (estrone sulfate/0.625 mg/d) had a small (0.8 percent) decrease in spine density at 24 months.
* The placebo group and the 0.3 mg (estrone sulfate) group loss bone mineral density.
* At 24 months, those women receiving HRT 0.3 mg/d had greater bone loss than the placebo group (−5.1 percent vs −3.6 percent).
* The placebo group did not lose as much bone density as was expected (1.8 percent annual loss).

Researchers' Comments: "This study support the findings ... that daily doses of less than 0.625 mg of conjugated estrogens were ineffective in preventing the loss of bone" (1983).

Participants and Methods: This two-year study (double blind) involved 120 postmenopausal women from three different study sites. The women were assessed for general health, medical conditions, reproductive history, blood chemistry, medications and estrogen use. Baseline information concerning alcohol, tobacco or coffee consumption was not obtained. The women were randomly assigned to one of four treatment groups: estrone sulfate (0.3 mg/d), estrone sulfate (0.625 mg/d), estrone sulfate (1.25 mg/d) or placebo. The women received HRT for 25 days monthly with six days off. All the subjects received 1.25 mg of calcium daily. Spine bone density was measured at 6, 12, 18 and 24 months. No significant differences in trabecular bone density were measured at baseline among the treatment groups.

► Herzberg M, Lusky A, Blonder J, and Frenkel Y.

The effect of estrogen replacement therapy on zinc in serum and urine. **Obstetrics and Gynecology,** June 1996; 87:1035–1039. **Type:** Experimental (clinical trial)

Focus: An investigation of the influence of HRT on blood and urinary zinc in postmenopausal women.

Conclusions: Women who received HRT had a decrease in zinc excretion after three months. The change was more noticeable in women with osteoporosis and elevated zinc excretion.

Findings:

• HRT reduced excretion of zinc, magnesium, *hydroxyproline* in those women who had elevated zinc excretion.
• At baseline, the values of most markers of bone turnover were higher in women with osteoporosis.
• Women with osteoporosis who received HRT had a decrease in zinc and magnesium excretion.
• Elevated zinc excretion associated with bone loss occurred in women in early menopause as well as women later in life.
• Women in the "normal" group who received HRT did not have a significant change in *zinc excretion.*

Researchers' Comments: "The results of our study suggest that zinc metabolism is intimately involved with bone metabolism and confirm previous data on a link between elevated zinc excretion and osteoporosis" (1039).

Participants and Methods: The study conducted from February 1991 to May 1993 involved thirty-seven postmenopausal women averaging 53.2 years in a menopause clinic in Israel. None of the women had received HRT and women was excluded for an abnormal pap smear, hypertension, liver disease, kidney disease, cardiovascular disease, diabetes, breast cancer or a thromboembolic condition. Treatment consisted of combined therapy estrogen (0.625 mg/d) + medroxyprogesterone acetate (5 mg/d). The estrogen was taken for 25 days, and the progestin for days 13–25. No treatment was taken for days 26–30 or 31. The women were also assessed for blood mineral content and bone mineral density. Zinc, magnesium, calcium, phosphate and alkaline phosphate levels were measured before and at six and twelve months of the study. Urine excretion of zinc, magnesium, calcium, phosphate and hydroxyproline was evaluated before HRT and at three, six and twelve months.

➤ Horsman A, Gallagher J, Simpson M, and Nordin B.

Prospective trial of oestrogen and calcium in postmenopausal women. *British Medical Journal*, September 1977; 2:789–792. **Type:** Experimental (clinical trial)

Focus: An examination of the effects of the HRT and calcium on bone loss in postmenopausal women.

Conclusions: HRT (*ethinyl estradiol*) prevents bone loss and calcium treatment retards bone loss in postmenopausal women. Estrogen appears to inhibit bone resorption.

Findings:
• Women who were in the untreated control group had bone loss during the study period.
• Women who received estrogen did not have bone loss.
• Bone loss in the calcium treated group was more than the estrogen treated group but less than the control group.
• At baseline, there was no significant difference in bone mineral density among the three groups.
• The control group lost bone mineral density from the forearm and *metacarpals* during the two-year trial.

Researchers' Comments: Although the mean time since the menopause in our patients was about six years, all the groups contained a high proportion of women within three years of menopause. This explains why our control group lost bone at a rate considerably higher than controls in previous series" (792).

Participants and Methods: Seventy-two postmenopausal women completed this two-year trial initiated in 1973. Fifty of the women who had completed the trial had received oophorectomies. Women were excluded from the study if they had spinal osteoporosis or any condition known to affect the rate of bone loss. Four groups comprised the study: controls (no treatment), estrogen treated group, calcium group and estrogen plus calcium treated group. The HRT group received ethinyl estradiol (25 or 50 μg daily for three weeks out of four). Women in the calcium group received two calcium gluconate tablets daily (about 800 mg of calcium). The control group did not receive a placebo. There was a high dropout rate in the fourth group so the researchers did not include data on this group in their report. All the participants were assessed for general health, reproductive status, medical conditions and medications and estrogen use. Bone loss was assessed at baseline and from four to six months using *densitometry* and morphometry.

▶ Horsman A, Jones M, Francis R, and Nordin C.

The effect of estrogen dose on postmenopausal bone loss, **The New England Journal of Medicine**, December 1983; 309:1405–1407. **Type:** Observational (cohort)

Focus: An evaluation of the effectiveness of estrogen (ethinyl estradiol) in preventing postmenopausal bone loss.

Conclusions: HRT (ethinyl estradiol) at higher daily doses (50 μg/d) was effective in preventing bone loss in postmenopausal women. The effect of ethinyl estradiol on bone loss is dose related.

Findings:

- Women who received HRT (ethinyl estradiol, 15 and 25 μg/d) neither gained nor lost bone mass.
- Low dosages of ethinyl estradiol (15 μg/daily or less) resulted in bone loss.
- Women who received ethinyl estradiol at higher doses (50 μg/d) had an increase in cortical bone mass.

Researchers' Comments: "It may be that the gap between the relatively small dose of estrogen that is required to control symptoms and the somewhat larger dose required for optimal bone effect could be bridged by combining a small dose of estrogen with a calcium supplement" (1407).

Participants and Methods: This study, initiated in 1973, involved 120 postmenopausal women (33 to 69 years) who were being treated with ethinyl estradiol at dosages of 5 to 50 μg/daily. The women were assessed for general health, medical conditions, estrogen use and reproductive history. Higher dosages employed cyclically, were used in the early 1970's before the risks of estrogen therapy were known. Later intermediate doses were used so the women would not be at an increased risk for adverse conditions. The effect of this treatment on cortical bone loss in the hand was measured by radiographic morphometry.

▶ Hutchinson T, Polansky S, and Feinstein A.

Postmenopausal estrogens protect against fractures of hip and distal radius. **The Lancet**, October 1979; 2:705–709. **Type:** Observational (case-control)

Focus: An investigation of the effect of HRT (estrogen) on hip and distal radius fractures in postmenopausal women.

Conclusions: HRT (unopposed estrogen) protects a woman against bone fractures. The data does not show the minimum dosage or duration of use required to have a positive effect.

Findings:

- Postmenopausal women who received HRT (unopposed estrogen) had a lower risk of hip and *distal radius* fractures than nonusers.
- *Perimenopausal* women who received HRT (unopposed estrogen) had a lower risk of hip and distal radius fracture than nonusers.
- Postmenopausal women who received HRT (unopposed estrogen) had a lower risk of hip and distal fracture than nonusers.
- Perimenopausal women who received HRT (unopposed estrogen) had a lower risk of hip and distal fracture than nonusers.
- X-rays indicated that osteoporosis was found in 32 percent of the fracture cases, and in 15 percent of the controls.

Researchers' Comments: "A mere six months of estrogen therapy cannot be regarded as sufficient to produce a protective effect, since we are not certain that the exposed women took estrogen for only six months. Many of these women, who are now in their 60s and 70s, could not remember how long they had taken estrogen, but were counted as exposed because they stated they had maintained it for a minimum of six months. These difficulties with detail of the remembered exposure also make it impossible to produce precise dose or duration curves" (707).

Participants and Methods: Participants in the study were 2609 female patients (40 years or more) who were admitted to the orthopedic service of Yale–New Haven Hospital between June 1974 and September 1977. The cases, 157 postmenopausal women (80 years or less) who had been admitted to the hospital with fractures of the hip or distal radius, were matched with controls admitted to the hospital for other conditions. The cases and controls were age and race matched but were differed in a number of variables: cases tended to be older at menopause, weighed less and drank more alcoholics than the control group. The controls were heavier than the cases. The women were assessed for estrogen uses (dose, duration and pattern) through medical records and patient interviews.

▶ **Kohrt W, Ehsani A, and Birge S.**

HRT preserves increases in bone mineral density and reduction in body fat after a supervised exercise program. *Journal of Applied Physiology,* January 1998; 84:1506–1512. **Type:** Experimental (clinical trial)

Focus: An investigation of the effect of HRT on bone mineral density in postmenopausal women when combined with exercise.

Conclusions: Use of HRT enhances the effect of exercise on bone mineral density and may prevent abdominal fat accumulation when coupled with exercise. Weight-bearing exercise increased bone mineral density in nonuser of HRT.

Results:

• HRT increased bone mineral density in postmenopausal women who exercised and this gain in bone mineral density was preserved even when exercise was decreased or stopped.

• HRT plus exercise was more effective at increasing bone mineral density then exercise or HRT alone.

• Postmenopausal women who did not receive HRT but participated in weight-bearing exercise had an increase in bone mineral density.

• Women who did not receive HRT lost bone mineral density when weight bearing exercise was decreased or stopped.

• HRT alone did not cause a decrease in either total or abdominal fat.

• HRT when coupled with exercise did not increase bone mineral density uniformly at all bone sites.

Researchers' Comments: "What remains perplexing is why the potentiating effect of estrogen on exercise-induced gains in BMD would be apparent for the whole body and some regional sites but not for others. Although the loading characteristics of the exercise program were sufficient to induce an increase in BMD of the femoral neck, there was no augmentation of BMD at that site by estrogen in the exercise + HRT group.... Further studies are clearly necessary to delineate the mechanisms by which exercise and estrogen regulate bone metabolism" (1510).

Participants and Methods: This small trial involved 54 postmenopausal women (60–72 years) who had not used estrogen for at least two years, were nonsmokers and had not participated in regular exercise. The women were assessed for general health, reproductive history, medical conditions, blood and urine profile, estrogen use, mammography and medications. Women were excluded from the study if they had medical conditions that contraindicated HRT or exercise. The treatment phase lasted for 11 months and the follow-up phase lasted for six months. The women were assigned to one of the following groups: controls (n=10); exercise alone (n=18); exercise + HRT (n=16) and HRT alone (n=10). HRT was combined therapy (estrogens, 0.625 mg/d + medroxyprogesterone acetate, 5mg/d). The exercise program involved two months of flexibility training followed by nine months of weight-bearing exercise (walking, jogging, stair climbing and descending). Three exercise sessions were required weekly, but the women were left to choose how much exercise they performed during the follow-up. The participants completed seven-day food records at the beginning and at the end of the treatment period and at the end of the follow-up phase. The calcium intake for the women was about 1500 mg/day. Bone mineral density of the total body, lumbar spine and proximal femur were measured using dual-energy, X-ray absorptiometry at three month intervals throughout the study.

➤ Komulainen M, Kroger H, Tuppurainen M, Heikkinen A, Alhava E, Hokanen R, Jurvelin J, and Saarikoski S.

Prevention of femoral and lumber bone loss with hormone replacement therapy and vitamin D-3 in early postmenopausal women: a population-based 5-year randomized trial. *Journal of Clinical Endocrinology and Metabolism*, February 1999; 84:546–552. **Type:** Experimental (clinical trial)

Focus: An examination to determine if low dose vitamin D supplementation in combination with long term sequential combined therapy (estrogen + progestin) has a positive impact on bone mineral density of the spine in early postmenopausal women.

Conclusions: HRT is effective at preventing bone loss, but vitamin D supplementation does not prevent bone loss in postmenopausal women.

Findings:

- Women who received combined therapy (estrogen + progestin) had a slight increase in bone mineral density of the spine (lumbar) of 0.2 percent based on intention to treat analysis.
- Women who received HRT plus vitamin D had a slight increase in bone mineral density of the spine of 0.9 percent based on intention to treat analysis.
- Women who received the placebo had a decrease in bone mineral density of the spine of 4.5 percent and women who received Vitamin D alone had a decrease in bone mineral density of the spine by 4.6 percent.
- All treatment groups had a loss of hip (femoral) bone mineral density: HRT group (−1.4 percent), HRT +Vitamin D group (−1.3 percent), Vitamin D group (−4.3 percent) and Placebo (−4.3 percent).
- Women who complied with the treatment for the entire study period (5 years) had the most significant bone mineral density in the spine (+1.5 percent for the HRT group; +1.8 percent for the HRT + vitamin D group)

Researchers' Comments: "In this study, the HRT effect was mainly obtained during the first 2.5 year and plateaued for the last 2.5 years" (550).

Participants and Methods: This five-year conducted in Finland was part of the larger Kuopio Osteoporosis Risk Factor and Prevention Study initiated in 1989. The participants, 464 postmenopausal women (47 to 56 years), were assessed for general health, lifestyle factors (diet, exercise, cigarette and alcohol consumption), medical conditions, reproductive history, medications and estrogen use. Women were excluded if they had a history of osteoporosis, cancer, vascular disease, medication-resistant hypertension. At baseline, 2.5 years and at the end of the five-year study each woman underwent bone mineral density tests using dual X-ray absorptiometry. At baseline, at the end of each study year and at the end of the study the women underwent gynecological examinations. The women were randomized into one of four treatment groups: HRT group (sequential combination of 2 mg estradiol valerate, days 1–21/1 mg cyproterone acetate daily), vitamin D-3 group (300 or 100 IU/d during the fifth year), HRT and vitamin D group, or placebo group.

> **Lindsay R, Aitken J, Anderson J, Hart D, MacDonald E, and Clarke A.**

Long-term prevention of postmenopausal osteoporosis by oestrogen. *The Lancet,* May 1976; 1:1038–1040. **Type:** Experimental (clinical trial)

Focus: An examination of the affect of estrogen on the prevention of osteoporosis in postmenopausal women.

Conclusions: HRT (estrogen) had beneficial short-term effects in slowing bone loss after menopause.

Findings:

- Women who received estrogen therapy (mestranol) from three to six years after their oophorectomies, had an increase in bone mineral density during the first three years of therapy, but thereafter there was no further increase in bone density.
- Bone loss occurs most rapidly three years after an oophorectomy but slows thereafter.
- The placebo group loss bone continuously except the period between 1.5 and 2 years after their oophorectomies.
- Women who received estrogen therapy (*mestranol*) had significantly lower hydroxyproline, *phosphate* and *alkaline phosphatase* levels than the placebo group.
- Women who received estrogen therapy (mestranol) had a reduction in

the calcium and hydroxyproline urinary levels significantly during the first three years of treatment.

Researchers' Comments: "We believe that oestrogen treatment is effective in preventing postmenopausal osteoporosis as measured by a reduction in bone mineral content. However, whether oestrogen given at this stage will prevent the clinical complications of osteoporosis, such as fractures of long bones and crush fractures of the spine, remains to be seen" (1040).

Participants and Methods: This five year trial (double blind) involved 63 women who had the ovaries surgically removed (oophorectomy) and were given estrogen replacement (mestranol/24.8 µg daily) or a placebo. The women were assessed for general health, reproductive status and medications. Biochemical markers of bone density (serum calcium, phosphate, alkaline phosphatase, urinary hydroxyproline) were measured at baseline and at yearly visits. Three study groups were formed based on the time after oophorectomy (two months, three years or six years). All the participants had their bone density (metacarpal) measured by photon absorptiometry every six months during the first three years and annually thereafter.

➤ **Lindsay R, MacLean A, Kraszewski A, Hart D, Clark A and Garwood J.**

Bone response to termination of oestrogen treatment. *The Lancet*, June 1978; 1:1325–1327. **Type:** Observational (cohort)

Focus: An examination of the effectiveness of oestrogen replacement in preventing bone loss.

Conclusions: HRT (estrogen therapy) is effective at preventing bone loss at least for eight years.

Findings:

- Bone loss may be most rapid the first three or four years after menopause or after an oophorectomy.
- Women who received the placebo initially had rapid bone loss (2.6 percent) annually; later this bone loss decreased to an average of (0.75 percent) annually.
- Women who received HRT (mestranol) for four years had no bone loss; however, upon withdrawal of estrogen therapy bone mineral density decreased at a rate of (2.5 percent) annually.
- Eight years after the initial therapy, women who had stopped HRT, had bone mineral density measurements similar to the placebo group.
- Fourteen women who had received estrogen for four years had no

bone loss until withdrawal of estrogen resulting in a 2.5 percent annual decrease in bone mineral density.

Researchers' Comments: "If we wish to prevent the increase in fracture incidence, how long should treatment last? If bone loss consequent on oestrogen removal is assumed to occur at the maximum rate and follow the pattern of post-oophorectomy bone loss ... reaching a maximum at 3–4 years—the 10 years of active oestrogen treatment after oophorectomy or the menopause will be needed to delay significantly the onset of an increase in fracture incidence" (1327).

Participants and Methods: The original group in this British study, 43 women who had their ovaries surgically removed, participated in a cohort study. Fourteen women were reviewed four years after withdrawal from HRT (mestranol). Another group of 14 women who had been given a placebo as part of the trial, and a third group of 15 women completed eight years of HRT (mestranol). Treatment (mestranol 27.6 μg/d) lasted for four years in two groups (placebo and mestranol), and for eight years in another mestranol group. The women were assessed for general health, medical conditions, medications, and reproductive history. This study was part of the follow-up to the original trial conducted in 1973. Bone mineral content of the hands were measured by photon absorptiometry.

▶ **Lindsay R, Hart D, and Clark M.**

The minimum effective dose of estrogen for prevention of postmenopausal bone loss. *Obstetrics and Gynecology*, June 1984; 63:759–763.
Type: Experimental (clinical trial)

Focus: An investigation to determine the minimum effective dosage of estrogen to protect against bone loss postmenopausal women.

Conclusions: Women who received conjugated estrogen of at least 0.625 mg/d were protected against bone loss. Lower doses of estrogen (less than 0.625 mg/d) were ineffective at protecting against bone loss.

Findings:

• Women who received conjugated estrogen of less than 0.625 mg/d were not protected against bone loss.

• Total serum calcium and phosphate were reduced in women who received conjugated estrogen (0.625 mg/d).

• Urinary calcium was reduced in women who received conjugated estrogen (0.625/1.25 mg/d).

• Hydroxyproline levels were reduced in women receiving conjugated estrogen (0.625/1.25 mg/d).

Researchers' Comments: "More information is required as to whether or not there is a synergistic effect between estrogen and calcium in protection against osteoporosis" (762).

Participants and Methods: The study was conducted for two years involving 108 women. Thirty women were allocated to one of four dosages of conjugated estrogen: 1.25, 0.625, 0.3 and 0.15 mg/d. The women were assigned to a treatment regimen randomly and prescribed nonmatching placebo tablets. All the participants were assessed for general health, medical conditions, medications and reproductive history. Laboratory tests were performed on the subjects at baseline and six month intervals. The women had their bone mineral content measured by photon absorptiometry. Urinary calcium and hydroxyproline were measured.

➤ **Michaëlsson K, Baron J, Farahmand B, Johnell O, Magnusson C, Persson P, Persson I, and Ljunghall S (for the Swedish Hip Fracture Study Group).**

Hormone replacement therapy and risk of hip fracture: population based case-control study. *British Medical Journal*, June 1998; 316:1858–1862. **Type:** Observation (case-control)

Focus: An investigation of the relationship between HRT and the risk of hip fracture.

Conclusions: In order for HRT to be effective in preventing hip fracture therapy must be continued for many years. Little protection against hip fractures remains after five years without HRT. Low dose estrogen or estradiol were not effective in preventing hip fractures. Women can begin receiving HRT several years after menopause without loss of fracture protection.

Findings:
• Women who received HRT estrogen alone had a decreased risk of hip fractures (**odds ratio:** 0.69 for users/1.00 for nonusers).
• Oral and transdermal HRT are equally effective in reducing the risk of hip fracture.
• Low dose conjugated estrogen (0.325 mg/d) or estradiol (1 mg/d) were not associated with a reduction in the risk of hip fractures.
• The minimum dose of estrogen effective in preventing bone loss in postmenopausal women is 2 mg/daily of estradiol or 0.625 mg/d of conjugated estrogen. Combined therapy (estrogen + progestin) had a better affect on bone density than estrogen.

Researcher's Comments: "The principal limitations of an observation study such as ours are possible confounding and measurement error as well as response biases.... A particular concern is that women who take hormone replacement therapy may have lower risk fractures for reasons other than the hormone replacement therapy" (1862).

Participants and Methods: The cases were 1327 women (50 to 81 years) with hip fractures who were identified through hospital discharge records and treated from October 1993 to February 1995 in six counties in Sweden. The controls were women born in Sweden who were randomly selected from the national, population register. Two controls were matched with every case according to age. The cases and controls were assessed through questionnaires for general health, medical history, lifestyle (diet, alcohol and cigarette consumption, physical activity) reproductive history and HRT (type, dosage, duration).

➤ **Naessen T, Berglund L, and Ulmsten U.**

Bone loss in elderly women prevented by ultralow doses of parenteral 17μ-estradiol. **American Journal of Obstetrics and Gynecology,** July 1997; 177:115–119. **Type:** Experimental (clinical trial)

Focus: An investigation of the effects of ultralow dose estradiol on bone mineral density and bone metabolism in postmenopausal women.

Conclusions: Ultralow doses of estradiol may prevent bone loss in women 60 years and older.

Findings:
• Forearm bone density increased in women who received HRT (estradiol) by 2.1 percent.
• Women who did not receive HRT had a decrease in forearm bone density by −2.7 percent.
• Biochemical markers of bone turnover (e.g., alkaline phosphatase) decreased in women who received estradiol.
• Women who did not receive HRT had no significant changes in markers of bone metabolism (e.g., alkaline phosphatase).
• Serum estradiol levels remained constant over time in both the HRT and no treatment groups.

Researchers' Comments: "The results from this short-term pilot study need therefore to be confirmed by studies with a longer duration or follow-up (more than 2 years) and including bone measurements at the spine and hip sites before this regimen can be recommended for prevention of osteoporosis" (118).

Participants and Methods: Thirty women (60 years or older) participated in this Swedish clinical trial lasting six months. The women were assessed for general health, medical conditions, reproductive status, estrogen use, biochemical markers of bone turnover and medications. The women were randomized to one of two treatment groups: vaginal ring releasing 17-ß estradiol or no treatment. Women with diseases or medications known to affect bone metabolism were excluded. An ultra low dose of 17-ß estradiol used for treatment of vaginal atrophy was given in a vaginal ring every third month.

➤ Prince R, Smith M, Dick I, Price R, Webb P, Henderson K, and Harris M.

Prevention of postmenopausal osteoporosis, a comparative study of exercise, calcium supplementation and hormone-replacement therapy. *The New England Journal of Medicine*, October 1991; 325:1189–1195.
Type: Experimental (clinical trial)

Focus: An investigation of how exercise, calcium and HRT affect bone mineral development and osteoporosis.

Conclusions: Postmenopausal women who have low bone mineral density can slow bone loss by exercising and taking calcium supplements or HRT. Exercise and HRT prevented less bone loss but also have more side effects than exercise plus calcium supplements.

Findings:
- Both exercise plus calcium supplementation and exercise plus HRT (combined therapy) were effective in slowing or stopping bone loss in women at increased risk for fractures.
- Exercise alone was generally not effective at preventing bone loss.
- Women who had a history of walking (moderate to brisk) for two hours per day had no bone loss in distal-forearm density.
- Women who exercised and received HRT had a 5.4 percent increase in bone density in the distal forearm.
- Women who exercised and received HRT had more vaginal bleeding and breast discomfort than the exercise group or calcium plus exercise group.

Researchers' Comments: "It may be appropriate to advise women with intermediate bone-density values to adopt the exercise and calcium regimen and to reserve estrogen for women with low bone density" (1195).

Participants and Methods: This two year clinical trial (double blind) in Australia involved women who were at increased risk of fracture because of low bone density. These women were postmenopausal (43 years or more). One hundred and twenty women participated in the trial and were randomly assigned to one of three study groups: group one—exercise alone, group two—exercise plus one gram of calcium lactate gluconate; group three—exercise plus continuous combined therapy (medroxyprogesterone acetate, 2.5 mg/d + estrogen, 0.625 mg/d for one month and then 1.25 mg/d estrogen for the remainder of the study period). The control group were women who had normal bone density. The exercise program involved one aerobics class weekly with a physiotherapist and two brisk 30 minute walks per week. The women were measured every three months for forearm bone density and the women were physically examined every six months during the two-year trial. A 24-hour urine sample, a fasting 2-hour urine sample for measuring (for calcium metabolism) and fasting blood sample were conducted at baseline and at intervals of six months during the trial. The women were also quantified (scored) according to reported symptoms.

➤ Recker R, Saville P, and Heaney R

Effects of Estrogens and Calcium Carbonate on Bone Loss in Postmenopausal Women. *Annals of Internal Medicine*, December 1977; 87:649–654. **Type:** Experimental (clinical trial)

Focus: An investigation of the effects of calcium supplements and HRT on bone mineral density in postmenopausal women.

Conclusions: Calcium carbonate supplements and estrogen therapy reduced bone loss in postmenopausal women. HRT prevented the greatest loss of bone mass, but it did not increase bone mass.

Findings:

• Women who received estrogen therapy or calcium carbonate supplements had less metacarpal bone loss than the control group.

• Women who received estrogen therapy during a two year period had 0.03696 mm average loss of cortical bone thickness.

• Women who received calcium carbonate during a two year period had a 0.05496 mm average loss of cortical bone thickness.

• Skeletal mass decreased by 0.15 percent per year in the hormone group, 0.22 percent per year in the calcium carbonate group and 2.88 percent in the control group.

• HRT (conjugated equine estrogen + methyltestosterone) did not increase bone mass.

Researchers' Comments: "Although these and other studies show that sex hormone treatment will minimize postmenopausal bone loss and a rational mechanism to explain this effect exists, it is difficult to decide which patients should be treated. It would seem unwise to subject the entire population of postmenopausal women to the risk of long-term sex hormone therapy to protect 25 percent or so that are at risk of developing symptomatic osteoporosis after age 65" (654).

Participants and Methods: The participants in this two-year study were 65 postmenopausal women (55–65 years) who were nuns belonging to a Catholic religious order with headquarters in Omaha, Nebraska. The women were assessed for general health, reproductive status, medical conditions, calcium balance and medications. They were randomized (not blinded) into three study groups: (1) the control group (no treatment) (2) conjugated equine estrogen (0.625 mg/d) plus *methyltestosterone* (5 mg/21 days of each month) (3) calcium carbonate (1200 mg/d). Bone mineral density was measured at baseline and at six month intervals using radiogrammetry, photon absorptiometry and X-ray densitometry.

> ### Riis B, Thomsen K, and Christiansen C.

Does Calcium Supplementation prevent postmenopausal bone loss? *The New England Journal of Medicine*, January 1987; 316:173–177. **Type:** Experimental (clinical trial)

Focus: An investigation of the effect of calcium supplementation of bone loss in postmenopausal women

Conclusions: Calcium supplements (dosages used) are not as effective as estrogen therapy for the prevention of early postmenopausal bone loss. Calcium supplements are more effective than no treatment.

Findings:
• Calcium supplements affected cortical bone but no effect on trabecular bone.
• Calcium supplements were not as effective as HRT (estrogen) for the prevention of early postmenopausal bone loss.
• The calcium-treated group had a much slower rate of bone loss in the *proximal forearm* than the placebo group.
• After 24 months, women receiving estrogen had a decrease in all the biochemical indicators of bone turnover (e.g., alkaline phosphatase, bone-Gla-protein, hydroxyproline).
• Calcium did not affect bone mass in the spine or in the *distal forearm*, areas of high trabecular bone content.

Researchers' Comments: "The bone mineral content in the distal forearm has been shown to correlate significantly with spinal bone mineral content" (176).

Subjects and Methods: This two-year study was part of a large double-blind, controlled trial conducted in Denmark from June 1983 to December 1985. The total number of participants was 270 postmenopausal women, with 43 women providing the data for this study. The women were assessed for general health, medical conditions, reproductive status and medication. All the women were free of any disease or condition known to influence calcium metabolism. The participants were randomized to one of three study groups: estradiol cream (3 mg/d combined with 200 mg of cyclic progesterone during the second year), oral calcium (2000 mg of calcium/d) and the placebo group (placebo cream + 2000 mg of calcium/d). All the women were examined every three months that included urine and blood analysis. Bone mineral content of the forearms was measured by *single-photon absorptiometry*. The bone mineral density of the spine and total skeleton was measured by *dual-photon absorptiometry*. Biochemical markers of bone turnover (alkaline phosphatase, Gla-protein, hydroxyproline) were also measured.

➤ Torgerson D and Bell-Syer S.

Hormone replacement therapy and prevention of nonvertebral fractures. *Journal of the American Medical Association*, June 2001; 285:2891–2897. **Type:** Statistical (meta-analysis)

Focus: A review of the randomized trials of HRT that have collected data on nonvertebral bone fractures.

Conclusions: Women who used HRT had a reduced risk of nonvertebral fractures. However, this effect was not found in older women receiving HRT.

Findings:
- Women who used HRT had a 27 percent reduction in *nonvertebral* fractures.
- Women who used HRT and were less than 60 years of age had more of a reduction in fractures than women over 60 years.
- Women less than 60 years who used HRT had a reduced risk of hip and wrist fractures (***relative risk:*** 0.45 for users/1.00 for nonusers).
- Women who started HRT before age 60 had a 35 percent reduction in nonvertebral fractures.

Researchers' Comments: "For women who started HRT before the age of 60 years and are still receiving treatment, observational data would suggest it is still effective; it is the age of starting therapy that our data would suggest is important" (2895).

Participants and Methods: This meta-analysis was prepared using MEDLINE, EMBASE, Science Citation Index and Cochrance Controlled Trials Register databases form 1997 to 2000. Older studies were also reviewed using systematic reviews. Pharmaceutical companies and researchers were also contacted to gain information from unpublished studies. The researchers identified 22 randomized trials of HRT with fracture data, including some unpublished data. The researchers included unblinded trials and trials without control groups. Most trials reported only certain outcomes (e.g., changes in bone density) and did not report fracture data. Trials were not included that only reported vertebral fractures. Only trials were included in which the women had been randomized to at least 12 months of treatment. Since fractures were included that resulted from any cause, the researchers noted that they may have included fractures caused by trauma or malignant disease not osteoporosis. Twenty-one of the twenty-two trials were designed to investigate the effects of estrogen on outcomes other than fracture and therefore did not enroll women identified as having osteoporosis.

> ### Villareal D, Binder E, Williams D, Schechtman K, Yarasheski K, and Kohrt W.

Bone mineral density response to estrogen replacement in frail elderly women. *Journal of the American Medical Association*, August 2001; 286:815–820. **Type:** Experimental (clinical trial)

Focus: An investigation of the effects of HRT on bone mineral density in frail, elderly women.

Conclusions: Elderly women who received HRT for nine months had a significant increase in bone mineral density.

Findings:
• Women who received HRT had a larger increase in bone mineral density of the lumbar spin than the placebo group.
• Women who received HRT for nine months had a 4.3 percent increase in bone mineral density in the lumbar spine.
• Women who received HRT for nine months had a 1.7 percent increase in bone mineral density in the hip.
• HRT reduced the serum levels of alkaline phosphatase, an indicator of bone loss.

Researchers' Comments: "Fracture risk in very old women is due to multiple factors in addition to low BMD, including sensory and neuromuscular impairments, medications and environmental hazards" (820).

Participants and Methods: This nine-month trial, conducted through the Washington University Older American Independence center (OAIC), involved 69 elderly women (75 years or more) from the area. Women were included in the study who were frail, as defined by the following three criteria: Low peak aerobic power, self-reported difficulty or need of assistance with some daily activities and moderate physical performance test scores. Women were excluded for prior estrogen use within the past year, a history of breast cancer or any other estrogen-dependent cancer, cancer within the previous five years, a history of thromboembolic disease, use of drugs that effect bone metabolism within the previous year and inconsistent thyroid medication within the previous three months. The women were assessed for general health, diet, calcium intake, estrogen use, medications, bone density (DEXA technology), serum markers of bone turn over (e.g., alkaline phosphatase) and medical conditions. The women were randomized to receive either HRT combined therapy, (conjugated estrogen, 0.625 mg/d + medroxyprogesterone acetate, 5mg/d for 13 days every third month) or placebo.

▶ Weiss N, Ure C, Ballard J, Williams A, and Daling J.

Decreased risk of fractures of the hip and lower forearm with postmenopausal use of estrogen. *The New England Journal of Medicine*, November 1980; 303:1195–1198. **Type:** Observational (case-control)

Focus: An examination of the relationship between HRT and the risk of fractures of the hip and lower forearm in postmenopausal women.

Conclusions: Women who received HRT (unopposed estrogen, 0.625 and 1.25 mg/d) for six years or more had about a 60 percent reduced risk of hip or forearm fracture compared to women who had not received HRT. Women who used HRT for a shorter time did not receive the same benefit.

Findings:

- HRT (unopposed estrogen) lowered the risk of hip fracture in women who used it for six or more years.
- HRT (unopposed estrogen) lowered the risk of forearm fracture in women who used it for six or more years.
- Conjugated estrogens of 1.25 mg/d or 0.625 mg/d were equally beneficial in preventing fractures.
- Women who used HRT (conjugated estrogens) had a lower risk of fractures than nonusers (**relative risk:** 0.38 for users for six or more years/1.00 for nonusers).
- A postmenopausal woman's risk of bone fractures increases with age.

Researchers' Comments: "If long-term estrogen use is assumed to lower the rate by 60 percent, a woman can expect to improve her chances by 0.3 to 3.0 per 1000 per year, depending on the type of fracture and her age. In terms of incidence itself, these projected reductions in risk are quantitatively smaller than the added incidence (5 to 25 per thousand per year) of endometrial cancer in such a woman if her uterus is intact" (1198).

Participants and Methods: The study, initiated from 1978 to 1979, involved 320 women with fractures of the hip or lower forearm, identified by Seattle-area orthopedic surgeons (through billing records and hospital-discharge indexes). The researchers interviewed 327 women who at the time of their fractures were 50 to 74 years. The cases were assessed for general health, medical conditions, fracture history, medications, estrogen use and reproductive history. Women were excluded from the study if they were institutionalized (e.g., nursing home), nonresidents of King County, Washington, had multiple fractures from a single accident or had pathologic fractures. The control group, 567 Caucasian women (50 to 74 years), had been interviewed during a household survey in King County in 1976, 1977 and 1997. The cases and controls were age and regionally matched.

➤ Wimalawansa S.

A four-year randomized controlled trial of hormone replacement and bisphosphonate, alone or in combination, in women with postmenopausal osteoporosis. *American Journal of Medicine,* March 1998; 104:219–226. **Type:** Experimental (clinical trial)

Focus: An investigation of the effectiveness of HRT plus etidronate on bone mineral density in postmenopausal women with osteoporosis.

Conclusions: HRT (combined therapy) plus *etidronate* was effective at improving bone mineral density in the spine and hip. Women who received HRT plus etidronate had higher bone mineral density in both the spine and hip than women who received HRT alone or etidronate alone.

Findings:

- Women who received HRT in combination with *bisphosphonate* (HRT plus etidronate) had increased bone mineral density in the lumbar spine by 10.4 percent in four years.
- Women who received HRT had increased bone mineral density in the spine by 7.0 percent in four years.
- Women who received Vitamin D and calcium lost 2.5 percent bone mineral density in spine in four years.
- Women who received etidronate alone had an increase in bone mineral density of the spine by 7.3 percent in four years but had a modest increase of only 0.9 percent at four years in hip bone density.
- All four treatment groups of women lost height during the follow-up period.

Researchers' Comments: "Although this study revealed a 10.5

percent increase of bone mass in the lumbar spine and 7 percent in the hip over the 4-year study period with combined therapy, it is unknown whether the increments of BMD observed will be continued over the long term, unless the cycle of resorption and formation is disrupted in favor of bone formation" (225).

Participants and Methods: This four year, small trial involved 72 Caucasian postmenopausal women (58 to 72 years) who had been diagnosed with osteoporosis. Women who had medical conditions or who had taken medications affecting calcium metabolism three years before the study were excluded. Women who had used HRT, anabolic steroids, glucocorticoids, calcitonin, fluoride, or bisphosphonates anytime during menopause were also excluded. The participants were assessed for general health, medical conditions, medications, reproductive history, HRT, and underwent mammography, blood chemistry screening and endometrial screening. The women were randomized into one of four treatment groups: control group (one gram of elemental calcium and 400 units of vitamin D/d); HRT group (conjugated estrogen, 0.625 mg/d + progestin, Norgestrel 150 μg/12 days each month), etidronate group (disodium etidronate, 400 mg for 14 days and intermittent cyclically administered every 12 weeks), and the combined therapy group (HRT and etidronate). All the women received one gram of elemental calcium and 400 units of vitamin D daily. Bone mineral density of the spine and hip was assessed using dual energy X-ray absorptiometry at baseline, year two and year four.

➤ Writing Group for the PEPI Trial.

Effects of hormone therapy on bone mineral density: results from the postmenopausal estrogen/progestin intervention (PEPI) trial. *Journal of the American Medical Association*, November 1996; 276:1389–1396.

Type: Experimental (clinical trial)

Focus: Part of the PEPI trial investigating the effects of HRT on bone mineral density in the spine and hip of postmenopausal women.

Conclusions: Unopposed estrogen (estrogen alone) increases bone mineral density in the spine and hip during three years of therapy. Combined therapy (estrogen + progestin) is not more effective than estrogen alone in maintaining or increasing bone mineral density.

Findings:
• Ethnicity, smoking, alcohol, calcium intake, physical activity and body mass did not modify the effect of estrogen on bone mineral density.
• Women receiving HRT gained bone mineral density; the placebo group lost bone mineral density.

- Age, initial bone mineral density and prior hormone use influenced the impact HRT had on bone mineral density.
- Combined therapy (estrogen + continuous progestin) increased bone mineral density, but it was not any better than estrogen alone.

Researchers' Comments: "Women who had never used hormones adhering to placebo had significantly less bone loss in the spine (−1.4 percent) and hip (−1.7 percent) than women who had previously used hormones (−4.6 percent and −2.8 percent respectively)" (1393).

Participants and Methods: The PEPI trial was a three-year, double blinded, study involving 875 women (45–64 years) recruited at seven clinical centers between 1989 and 1991. The main purpose of the trial was to study the effects of HRT on heart disease. A second goal was to ascertain the effects of HRT on bone mineral density at specific bone sites. The women were assessed for lifestyle characteristics (smoking, alcohol consumption, calcium intake and physical activity), general health, medical conditions, medications, estrogen use, reproductive history and blood chemistry profile. Bone mineral density was measured using dual-energy X-ray absorptionmetry at 12 months and 36 months. The women were randomized into one of five treatment groups: (1) placebo (2) conjugated equine estrogen, 0.625 mg/d (3) conjugated equine estrogen, 0.625 mg/d + medroxyprogesterone acetate, 10 mg for days 1 through 12 (4) conjugated equine estrogen, 0.625 mg/d + medroxyprogesterone acetate, 2.5 mg/d (5) conjugated equine estrogen, 0.625 mg/d + micronized progesterone, 200 mg for days 1 through 12.

5

Ovarian Cancer

Ovarian cancer is the most common fatal gynecologic malignancy and rates fifth in its incidence in white women (15.6 per 100,000). Women who live in industrial countries are at a higher risk for the disease. Although curable if found early, most often it is discovered in its later stages when it has metastasized to other organs because the symptoms of the disease are so vague. Three types of types of ovarian cancer are epithelial, germ cell and stromal tumors. Epithelial ovarian cancer, the most common form, originates in the cells covering the surface of the ovary. Epithelial carcinomas are typed as serous, mucinous, endometroid, Brenner or clear cell tumors. Epithelial tumors are classified as benign, borderline malignant or malignant. Germ cell tumors start in the eggs and stromal tumors, which are uncommon, arise from supportive tissue. Five percent of cases may be genetically related (BRCA genes) and the disease occurs most often after menopause in the seventh decade. It is the most frequent cause of cancer death in women in the United States with a 30 percent five-year survival rate. Lifetime risk estimates for ovarian cancer for women in the general population are 1.7 percent (17 out of 1,000) will get ovarian cancer. Women who carry mutated BRCA1 or BRCA2 genes have a 16 to 60 percent chance of developing ovarian cancer (160–600 out of 1,000). (http://www.nci.nih.gov; http://www.seer.cancer.gov)

The Causes of Ovarian Cancer Are Unknown

Years of ovulation damaging the surface epithelium of the ovary and repeated exposure to estrogen may be the causes of ovarian cancer. Obesity, early menarche, late menopause, exposure to talcum powder, asbestos and industrial toxins, nulliparity, Jewish descent (Eastern European), infertility, infertility drugs and estrogen therapy have been associated with an increased risk of ovarian cancer, but different studies often yielded conflicting results. Evidence for dietary causes of the disease is inconclusive, although a reduced risk of ovarian cancer is associated with intake of antioxidants and low-fat milk products (Fleischauer et al., 2001; Goodman et al., 2002) Mutations in BRCA genes have been identified in women with a family history of ovarian cancer. The lifetime risk of developing the disease in this group can be as high as fifty percent. A serum tumor marker using a protein called CA-125 is often used to help diagnose the disease. It is elevated in about eighty percent of the women who have epithelial ovarian cancer. However, it is not specific only to ovarian cancer and can be elevated for other reasons resulting in false-positives. Tumor markers are also useful for assessing response to therapy. Once diagnosed treatment often involves extensive pelvic surgery, and chemotherapy if metastases have occurred. Future treatment may entail gene therapy and tumor-toxic antibody therapy.

HRT and Ovarian Cancer

The relationship between HRT and the development of ovarian cancer is unclear. Many earlier studies found no association between HRT and ovarian cancer (Annegers et al., 1979; Hildreth et al., 1981; Hartge et al., 1988). Later studies have found a relationship (Rodriguez et al., 2001; Lacey et al., 2002; Garg et al., 1998). Limited data is available about the effects of between combined therapy on the development of ovarian cancer. Earlier studies evaluated estrogen alone and ovarian cancer. Ovarian cancer takes many years to develop and has the highest prevalence in women over 70. Combined therapy has not been used by women long enough to evaluate conclusively the relationship between estrogen plus progestin and ovarian cancer. Clinical Trials and observational studies using combined therapy are needed to provide more data and answer more questions.

Preventing Ovarian Cancer

Routine pelvic exams and especially pelvic ultrasound examinations are important, but are not perfect screening tools. Ovarian cancer does not present women with obvious symptoms. Most women with the disease report vague, nonspecific abdominal symptoms such as pain, pelvic pressure, low back discomfort, mild nausea, feeling full immediately after eating, constipation and gas, abnormal uterine bleeding. Therefore, diagnosing this cancer early is difficult. Preventive measures may include blocking ovulation by breast feeding and using oral contraceptives, carefully evaluation hormone use and having children (Lacey et al 2002; Rodriguez 2001; Whittemore et al., 1993). Tubal ligation also has been found to decrease a woman's risk of the disease. Women who have a family history of the disease can have genetic screening for the BRCA genes to assess their risk. In some cases, these women may decide to have their ovaries removed (prophylactic oophorectomy).

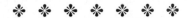

➤ **Annegers J, Strom H, Decker D, Dockerty M, and O'Fallon W.**

Ovarian cancer, incidence and case-control study. *Cancer,* February 1979; 43:723–729. **Type:** Observational (case-control)

Focus: An investigation of the incidence and risk factors of *ovarian cancer.*

Conclusions: Nulliparity was the only significant risk factor for ovarian cancer.

Findings:

• No major risk factors for ovarian cancer were identified except nulliparity.

• Long- term use of HRT (conjugated estrogen) was not associated with an increased risk of ovarian cancer.

• Women who had hysterectomies, even with preservation with one or both ovaries, had a lower risk of ovarian cancer.

• No increased risk of ovarian cancer was associated with obesity or prior use of estrogen.

• No association was found for age at menopause and ovarian cancer.

Researchers' Comments: "Long-term use of conjugated estrogens was not found to be associated with ovarian *carcinoma* in a population where a study utilizing the same methodology did find a highly significant association between endometrial carcinoma and long-term use of conjugated estrogen" (724).

Participants and Methods: The cases for this study were obtained using medical records (1935 through 1974) of the Rochester project at the Mayo Clinic in Rochester, Minnesota. The participants, 116 cases diagnosed with epithelial ovarian cancer, were age-matched with 464 controls. The controls were women who had been seen at the clinic for various conditions (emergency-room visits, general medical conditions, eye and dental exams). All the women were assessed for medical history, reproductive history and hormone use. The researchers also gathered data on ovarian cancer rates in Rochester from 1937 to 1974.

➤ Cramer D, Hutchison G, Welch W, Scully R, and Ryan K.

Determinants of ovarian cancer risk. I. Reproductive experiences and family history. *Journal of the National Cancer Institute*, October 1983; 71:711–716. **Type:** Observation (case-control)

Focus: An investigation of the effects of family history and reproductive history on the risk of ovarian cancer.

Conclusions: HRT (estrogen) was associated with an increased risk of ovarian cancer particularly in women who had used estrogen cyclically. Pregnancy has a protective effect against ovarian cancer.

Findings:

• Ever use of HRT was associated with an increased risk of ovarian cancer (**relative risk estimate**: 1.56 for users of conjugated estrogens/1.00 for nonusers).

• Women who used HRT (estrogen) for one year or less or five or more years had an increased risk of ovarian cancer.

• Women who had ovarian cancer had more frequently used HRT (estrogen) cyclically than controls.

• Women who had ovarian cancer had a higher number of relatives who had cancer of the lung, colon, ovary or prostate gland than controls.

• *Parity* was associated with a reduced risk of ovarian cancer and the risk decreased with increasing number of births.

Researchers' Comments: "We also observed excess risk of borderline statistical significance for women who used menopausal estrogens in cyclic fashion compared to continuous use and in women who had used the drug for more than 5 years" (715).

Participants and Methods: The cases were 215 Caucasian women (average age 53.2 years) who had been diagnosed with epithelial ovarian cancer from 1978 to 1981 in Massachusetts. The controls, selected from residency lists, were matched with cases by age, race and residency. The women were assessed for general health, family medical history, medical conditions, reproductive history, estrogen use and medications. Of the cases, 36.3 percent were premenopausal compared to 40.0 percent of the controls.

➤ Eeles R, Tan S, Wiltshaw E, Fryatt I, A'Hern R, Shepherd J, Harmer C, Blake P, and Chilvers C.

Hormone replacement therapy and survival after surgery for ovarian cancer. **British Medical Journal**, February 1991; 302:259–262. **Type:** Observational (case-control)

Focus: An evaluation of the effects of HRT on survival of women who have undergone an oophorectomy due to ovarian cancer.

Conclusions: HRT was not associated with an adverse effect on the survival of women with ovarian cancer.

Findings:

• No significant difference in survival between women who received HRT and those who did not, based on analysis of other survival related variables (e.g., stages of cancer, differentiation of tumors, histological results).

• Disease free survival time was not significantly different between the women who received HRT and nonusers (**relative risk estimate:** 0.90 for users/1.00 for nonusers).

• Women who had ovarian cancer and received HRT had a lower risk of mortality than nonusers (**relative risk estimate:** 0.73 for users/1.00 for nonusers).

• Combined therapy (estrogen + progestin) or estrogen alone were similar in their effects on patient survival.

• The group receiving HRT had a higher percentage of younger patients with early stage disease and more differentiated tumors.

Researchers' Comments: "There are two possible sources of bias in patients who do not start to receive the treatment until after the base time for the survival analysis (in this case base time was presentation at the hospital). Firstly, the effect, if any, will be present only after the date that hormone replacement therapy was first given. Secondly, patients have to survive long enough to develop menopausal symptoms and ask for hormone replacement therapy; hence those who do not live long after diagnosis would tend not to have received it, and this would give *spurious* positive survival effect for those receiving it. To overcome any bias due to these sources of error we applied two different methods of survival analysis...." (260)

Participants and Methods: The cases and controls were 373 women (50 years or less), diagnosed with epithelial ovarian cancer and underwent *bilateral salpingo-oophorectomies* between 1972 and 1988 in a British hospital in London. This study group was derived obtained using a hospital database. The women were assessed for general health, medical conditions, reproductive status, estrogen use (type and dosage) and medications. Women with ovarian cancer who did not receive hormone replacement after diagnosis formed the control group. The researchers, used a Landmark Method which employs an arbitrary point in time after the base time of analysis and considers only women who do not die before that time. The data compared women who had used HRT in the first year after diagnosis compared with women who did not use HRT within the first year of diagnosis. Seventy-eight patients had received HRT; 65 were given the treatment at the hospital outpatient visits and 13 had been started on HRT by their physicians. HRT consisted of estrogen alone (Premarin, 0.625 mg/d), combined therapy (Premarin, 0.625 mg/d + Norgestrel, 0.5 mg/d), progestin alone and testosterone alone. Ninety-five percent of the patients had started HRT within three years. Follow-up time ranged from less than one month to eighteen years.

▶ Garg P, Kerlikowske K, Subak L, and Grady D.

Hormone replacement therapy and the risk of epithelial ovarian carcinoma: a meta-analysis. **Obstetrics and Gynecology**, September 1998; 92:472–479. **Type:** Statistical (meta-analysis)

Focus: An investigation of the risk of invasive ovarian cancer in women who use HRT.

Conclusions: Long term use of HRT is associated with an increased risk of developing ovarian cancer.

Findings:

- Ever use of HRT was associated with an increased risk of ovarian cancer (**odds ratio:** 1.15 for users/1.00 for nonusers).
- Women who used HRT for ten years or more had an increased risk of ovarian cancer (**odds ratio:** 1.27 for users/1.00 for nonusers).
- No trend of increasing risk was associated with increasing duration of HRT use.
- Women who used HRT for one year or less had a slight increased risk of ovarian cancer (**odds ratio:** 1.12 for users/1.00 for nonusers).
- Inclusion of studies that had subjects with borderline tumors did significantly affect the result of this study.

Researchers' Comments: "Even a small increase in risk of ovarian cancer among women who use HRT is of concern because the disease is often incurable" (477).

Participants and Methods: This meta-analysis was based on research on HRT and Ovarian cancer from 1966 to 1997. The information was obtained through MEDLINE, bibliographies and consulting experts.

Three hundred and twenty-seven studies were reviewed but nine studies provided information of the risk of ovarian cancer in ever users of HRT. Nine studies were the focus. These nine observational studies age-matched cases and controls, had age-adjusted results and excluded women who had bilateral oophorectomies. Data was obtained about the type of study, the source of controls, histology or tumors, reproductive history and estrogen use (type, dosage, duration). HRT included estrogen alone therapy or combined therapy (estrogen + progestin).

➤ Harris R, Whittemore A, Itnyre J, and the Collaborative Ovarian Cancer Group.

Characteristics relating to ovarian cancer risk: Collaborative analysis of 12 US case-control studies (Part II: Epithelial tumors of low malignant potential in white women). **American Journal of Epidemiology**, November 1992; 136:1204–1211. **Type:** Statistical (meta-analysis)

Focus: An examination of the risk factors for *epithelial ovarian tumors* and a comparison of the risk factors for invasive ovarian epithelial cancer and epithelial ovarian tumors.

Conclusions: Women who have used fertility drugs have higher risk of non-invasive epithelial ovarian tumors.

Findings:
- Women who had used HRT (estrogen) generally did not have an increased risk of epithelial ovarian tumors; however, women who had used estrogen for one year or five to nine years had a slight increased risk (**odds ratio:** 1.30 for users/1.00 for nonusers).
- Duration of estrogen use was not associated with an increased risk of ovarian cancer.
- Nulliparous women had a higher risk of epithelial ovarian tumors than women who had given birth.
- Women who had fertility problems or who had used fertility drugs had an increased risk of epithelial ovarian tumors.
- Oral contraceptive use was associated with a decreased risk of epithelial ovarian tumors.
- Increased risk was associated with obesity.

Researchers' Comments: "Similarities between the present findings for epithelial ovarian tumors of low malignant potential and the findings of part II for invasive epithelial cancers strengthen the inferences for both and suggest that the two types of cancer have similar etiologies" (1210).

Participants and Methods: The data for this meta-analysis was obtained from nine case-control studies conducted in the United States from 1974 to 1986. This analysis was part of a larger meta-analysis of 12 case-control studies of ovarian cancer risks. Four of the studies were hospital based using hospital controls and five of the studies were population based using random population controls. The participants were 327 Caucasian women diagnosed with epithelial ovarian cancer of low malignant potential. This reports presents two analyses of this study group. One analysis deals with women with tumors of low malignant potential compared with controls; the other analysis examines characteristics of women with these borderline tumors compared with women with invasive tumors.

➤ **Hartge P, Hoover R, McGowan L, Lesher L, and Norris H.**

Menopause and ovarian cancer. *American Journal of Epidemiology*, May 1988; 127:990–998. **Type:** Observational (case-control)

Focus: An investigation of the impact of menopause on the incidence and risk of ovarian cancer

Conclusions: Women who have had hysterectomies with intact ovaries, or women who have used HRT (estrogen) have a reduced risk of ovarian cancer.

Findings:

• Women who had ever used HRT (estrogen) had a 40 percent reduction in the risk of ovarian cancer (*rate ratio estimate:* 0.60 for users/1.00 for nonusers).

• Women who had used HRT (estrogen) for less than one month had an increased risk of ovarian cancer (*rate ratio estimate:* 2.00 for users/1.00 for nonusers).

• Women who had a hysterectomy resulting in a surgical menopause had 30 percent reduction in the risk of ovarian cancer.

• Later age at menopause was not related to an increased risk of ovarian cancer.

• Hot flashes were associated with an increased risk of ovarian cancer.

• Women who experienced cramps during menopause had a lower risk of ovarian cancer.

Researchers Comments: "The overall protective effect estimated for menopausal estrogen use varied slightly according to whether other risk factors were present, with the protection generally being more marked in the groups at lower risk of ovarian cancer.... The protective effect was absent in blacks" (996).

Participants and Methods: This study, conducted in Washington,

D.C. from 1978 to 1981, involved 296 women (20 to 79 years) diagnosed with epithelial ovarian cancer. The cases included women with tumors of low malignant potential and malignant tumors. The controls, 343 women selected from hospital discharge lists, were matched with cases according to age, ethnicity, hospital, and date of discharge. The women were assessed for general health, tobacco and alcohol consumption, medical conditions, reproductive history, medications and estrogen use (type, duration). Twelve per cent of the cases and 14 per cent of the controls were black and the other participants were Caucasian. Sixty-eight per cent of the HRT users used conjugated estrogen (Premarin). The average age for diagnosis for cases was 54.4 years and 54.7 years for controls.

> **Hildreth N, Kelsey J, LiVolsi V, Fischer D, Holford T, Mostow E, Schwartz P, and White C.**

An epidemiologic study of epithelial carcinoma of the ovary. **American Journal of Epidemiology**, September 1981; 114:398–405. **Type:** Observational (case-control)

Focus: The identification of the risk factors associated with epithelial carcinoma of the ovary.

Conclusions: Prior use of postmenopausal estrogens did not increase the risk of *epithelial ovarian cancer*. Oral contraceptive use may be protective against ovarian cancer.

Findings:
* Women who had never married had a higher risk of ovarian cancer (**odds ratio:** 1.40).
* Jewish women had higher risk of ovarian cancer than non–Jewish women (**odds ratio:** 1.70).
* Women who were nulliparous had a higher risk of ovarian cancer (**odds ratio:** 1.70).
* Women who had a late menopause after age 50 had an increased risk of ovarian cancer (**odds ratio:** 2.90).
* Breast feeding did not alter the risk of ovarian cancer but use of oral contraceptives might be protective against ovarian cancer.
* HRT (estrogen) ever use was not associated with an increased risk of ovarian cancer.

Researchers' Comments: "Reproductive variables appear to play a role in the etiology of ovarian cancer, although the specific underlying mechanism, which is probably hormonal, is unknown" (403).

Participants and Methods: The data for this study was collected between July 1977 and March 1979. The cases were Caucasian women (45–74 years) admitted to seven Connecticut hospitals with a diagnosis of epithelial ovarian cancer. The controls, women admitted to the surgical services of the same hospitals for a variety of conditions, were age-matched with the cases. The women were assessed for general health, tobacco use, medical conditions, family history of cancer, reproductive history, medications and estrogen use. Women were excluded from the study if they had a previous diagnosis of breast cancer or other reproductive system cancer. Controls were excluded if they had their ovaries removed, were not residents of Connecticut or had a different racial background than the cases.

➤ Kaufman D, Kelly J, Welch W, Rosenberg L, Stolley P, Warshauer M, Lewis J, Woodruff J, and Shapiro S.

Noncontraceptive estrogen use and epithelial ovarian cancer. *American Journal of Epidemiology*, December 1989; 130:1142–1151. **Type:** Observational (case-control)

Focus: An investigation of the relation of HRT (estrogen alone and combined therapy) to the development of epithelial ovarian cancer.

Conclusions: HRT (estrogen alone) was associated with a slight increased risk of epithelial ovarian cancer but combined therapy was not associated with an increased risk. Long-term users estrogen alone therapy had an increased risk of ovarian cancer.

Findings:

- Women who had ever used estrogen alone had a slight increase in risk of epithelial ovarian cancer (*relative risk estimate:* 1.10 for users/1.00 for nonusers).
- Women who had ever used combined therapy (estrogen + progestin or estrogen + testosterone) had a decreased risk of epithelial ovarian cancer (*relative risk estimate:* 0.70 for users/1.00 for nonusers).
- Women who had used estrogen alone for more than 10 years had an increased risk of epithelial ovarian cancer (*relative risk estimate:* 1.60 for users/1.00 for nonusers).
- Women who used unopposed estrogens for five to nine years before being diagnosed with epithelial ovarian cancer had an increased risk of this cancer (*relative risk estimate:* 2.70 for users/1.00 for nonusers).
- Relative risk was not dose related; however, women who received 1.25 mg/daily or 0.3 mg /daily (conjugated estrogens) had an increased risk

of epithelial ovarian cancer (***relative risk estimate:*** 3.20 for users of 0.3 mg/daily, based on four cases/2.40 for users of 1.25 mg/daily based on 15 cases).

• Women who used estrogen had an increased risk of ovarian cancer, undifferentiated cell type (***relative risk estimate:*** 3.60 for users/ 1.00 for nonusers).

Researchers' Comments: "Given the lethality of ovarian cancer, the common use of estrogens by postmenopausal women and the lack of clarity in the results of endometrioid, undifferentiated, and other cell types, it is important to conduct studies with sufficient data to allow detailed analysis of each type" (1151).

Participants and Methods: This study was based on interviews conducted from September 1976 to October 1976, from hospitals in California, Canada and Israel. The cases, 377 women (18 to 69 years) diagnosed with ovarian cancer, were assessed for general health, medical conditions, reproductive history, estrogen use (type/dosage), medication history, alcohol and tobacco use. Details of the cases' diagnoses (e.g., histology classification) were obtained from hospital records and pathology slides were obtained for 57 percent of the cases allowing cell type classification. The control group, 2,030 women aged matched with cases, were female patients who had been hospitalized for nonmalignant conditions. HRT was primarily conjugated estrogen with various dosages (0.3 mg/d, 0.625 mg/d, 1.25 mg/d).

▶ **Lacey J, Mink P, Lubin J, Sherman M, Troisi R, Hartge P, Schatzkin A, and Schairer C.**

Menopausal hormone replacement therapy and risks of ovarian cancer. *Journal of the American Medical Association*, July 2002; 288: 334–341. **Type:** Observational (cohort)

Focus: An investigation of the association between HRT and the development of ovarian cancer.

Conclusions: Women who used HRT (estrogen alone) had an increased risk of ovarian cancer, especially long-term use (ten years or more). Short-term use of combined therapy (estrogen + progestin) was not associated with an increased risk of ovarian cancer. The association between the use of combined therapy and the development of ovarian cancer warrants more research.

Findings:

• Ovarian cancer risk decreased with the increased parity, oral contraceptive use and hysterectomy, but no association was found between age at menopause and BMI (body mass index) and the development of ovarian cancer.

- Women who received HRT (estrogen alone) had an increased risk of ovarian cancer (*relative risk:* 1.60 for users/1.00 for nonusers).
- Longer duration of estrogen use was associated with an increased risk of ovarian cancer (*relative risk:* 10 to 19 years, 1.80 for users/1.00 for nonusers/20 or more years, 3.20 for users/1.00 for nonusers).
- Increased risk of ovarian cancer was associated with HRT use in women who had hysterectomies and those who did not.
- Short-term (two years or less) use of combined therapy (estrogen + progestin) did not significantly increase a woman's risk of ovarian cancer (*relative risk:* 1.60 for users/1.00 for nonusers) and use of combined therapy (two or more years) did not increase a woman's risk of ovarian cancer (*relative risk:* 0.80 for users/1.00 for nonusers). However, the association was not clear since the data was only based on 18 women who used combined therapy and developed ovarian cancer.
- Women who had used estrogen alone therapy, but changed to combined therapy, had an increased risk of ovarian cancer (*relative risk:* 1.50 for users/1.00 for users).

Researchers' Comments: "Declining ERT use in the late 1970s reduced the number of potential long-term users and may have prevented earlier studies from detecting an association with ovarian cancer, which develops over many years" (340).

Participants and Methods: The researchers analyzed the follow-up data from the Breast Cancer Detection Demonstration Project follow-up study. The data was obtained during the follow-up period from 1979 to 1998. The BCDDP, a mammography screening program conducted at 29 U.S. centers between 1973 and 1980 by the American Cancer Society and the National Cancer Institute. In 1979, the NCI initiated a follow-up study of 64,182 of the original 283,222 participants. The BCDDP follow-up study consisted of four phases involving health assessment, oral interviews and questionnaires. The women were assessed for menopausal status, general health, medical conditions, medications, estrogen use (type/duration), risk factors, demographic data, height and weight. Women (12,581) were excluded because of the following conditions or status: bilateral oophorectomy, death, breast cancer before the follow-up. Analysis included 44,247 participants who completed phase I and 37,657 women who completed phase 2, 3 and 4 questionnaires. The final analysis included 329 women who developed ovarian cancer identified from medical records, registry data, self-reporting and death certificates. Follow-up time was an average of 13.4 years and the average age at the start of follow-up was 56.6 years.

Most of the HRT users questioned after 1992 used conjugated equine estrogens (0.625 mg/d) and medroxyprogesterone acetate (2.5 mg, 5.0 mg, 10.0 mg).

➤ **Polychronopoulou A, Tzonou A, Hsieh C, Kaprinis G, Rebelakos A, Toupadaki N, and Trichopoulos D.**

Reproductive variables, tobacco, ethanol, coffee and *somatometry* as risk factors for ovarian cancer. *International Journal of Cancer*, September 1993; 55:402–407. **Type:** Observational (case-control)

Focus: An investigation of variables and their association with ovarian cancer.

Conclusions: No consistent association was found for ovarian cancer and consumption of alcohol, coffee and tobacco. Nor was there an increased risk of ovarian cancer based on occupation or reproductive history (age of menarche /abortions). Oral contraceptives were associated with a lower risk of ovarian cancer, and HRT was associated with an increased risk of ovarian cancer.

Findings:
- Postmenopausal women who had used HRT (estrogen) had an elevated risk of ovarian cancer (***rate ratio estimate:*** 5.73 for users/1.00 for nonusers).
- Diabetes Mellitus was associated with an increased risk of ovarian cancer.
- Weight was weakly associated with an increased risk of ovarian cancer.
- Women who have given birth have a lower risk of ovarian cancer than nulliparous women.
- Miscarriages but not induced abortions were associated with ovarian cancer.
- The older a woman was at menopause, the greater was her risk of ovarian cancer.

Researchers' Comments: "Late age at menopause has been found to increase the risk of ovarian cancer in most European studies ... but not in most American investigations ... the reason for the discrepancy is not clear, although the widespread use of menopausal estrogens among American women could be a (partial) explanation" (406).

Participants and Methods: This study conducted from June 1989 to March 1991 involved 189 women (75 years or less) from Athens, Greece who had surgery for epithelial cancer in two major hospitals. The control group, 200 female residents of Athens with no history of cancer or oophorectomy, were visitors of patients hospitalized at the same time and in the same wards as the cancer patients. All participants were assessed for general health, medical history, reproductive history, medications, estrogen use, alcohol, tobacco and coffee consumption.

> **Purdie D, Green A, Bain C, Siskind V, Ward B, Hacker N, Quinn M, Wright G, Russell P, and Susil B (for the Survey of Women's Health Study Group).**

Reproductive and other factors and risk of epithelial ovarian cancer: an Australian case-control study. *International Journal of Cancer*, September 1995; 62:678–684. **Type:** Observational (case-control)

Focus: An examination of the incidence and risk factors for ovarian cancer in a cohort of Australian women.

Conclusions: No association was found between the development of ovarian cancer and the use of HRT (estrogen), menstrual history or terminated or incomplete pregnancy. Smoking, use of talc powder, high body mass index and family history of ovarian cancer were associated with an increased risk of ovarian cancer.

Findings:
- The more pregnancies a woman had, the lower her risk of ovarian cancer.
- Oral contraceptive use was associated with a lower risk of ovarian cancer.
- Tubal ligation was associated with a lower risk of ovarian cancer.
- Women with hysterectomies, had a lower risk of ovarian cancer.
- HRT was not significantly associated with an increased risk of ovarian cancer (**odds ratio:** 1.03 for users/1.00 for nonusers).
- Women with a family history of ovarian cancer had an elevated risk of ovarian cancer

Researchers' Comments: "The theory that incessant *ovulation* is a factor in the development of ovarian cancer ... is supported by some but not all, evidence from epidemiological studies. Reductions in risk associated with pregnancy and oral contraceptive use are the main factors that support the hypothesis as ovulation ceases during these times. In the present study we conclusively found that childbirth and OCP [oral contraceptive pill] use were associated with reduced risk of disease and that risk decreased with increased duration of OCP use and increased parity, which support the hypothesis. Other protective factors, such as hysterectomy and tubal ligation, do not appear relevant to the incessant ovulation theory as ovulation would not normally be suppressed after these surgeries" (683).

Participants and Methods: The cases were 824 women (18 to 79 years) diagnosed with ovarian cancer in three Australian states from 1990 to 1993. The controls were 860 women selected randomly from the electorate and age-matched with cases. The women were assessed for demographic characteristics, dietary and environmental factors general health, medical condition, reproductive history and estrogen use.

➤ Rodriguez C, Calle E, Coates R, Miracle-McMahill H, Thun M, and Heath C.

Estrogen Replacement therapy and fatal ovarian cancer. **American Journal of Epidemiology**, May 1995; 141:828–835. **Type:** Observational (cohort)

Focus: An investigation of the relation between short-term and long-term use of HRT and fatal ovarian cancer rates between perimenopausal and postmenopausal women.

Conclusions: Long-term use HRT (estrogen) increases the risk of fatal ovarian cancer.

Findings:

- Women who had used HRT had an increased risk of fatal ovarian cancer rate (*rate ratio:* 1.15 for users/1.00 for nonusers.
- Long-term users of HRT (6–10 years) had an increased risk of fatal ovarian caner (*rate ratio:* 1.71 for users/1.00 for nonusers).
- An increase in fatal ovarian cancer was associated with years of use in both current and former users.
- A decreased risk of ovarian cancer was associated with a late age at *menarche,* and use of oral contraceptives, but no other variables were associated with a statistically significant increase or decrease in ovarian cancer.
- Former users of HRT (estrogen) had a slight increased risk of ovarian cancer (*rate ratio:* 1.11 for users/1.00 for nonusers).

Researchers' Comments: "The findings from this study may not be generalized to today's estrogen replacement therapy users; the normal dose for estrogen replacement therapy was 1.25 mg prior to 1978, but currently it is 0.625 mg" (833).

Participants and Methods: The participants in this cohort study, conducted from 1982 to 1989, were 240,073 peri- and postmenopausal women recruited from the Cancer Prevention Study II, a prospective mortality study of 1.2 million US men and women initiated by the American

Cancer Society in 1982. Women were excluded if they had a history of cancer, hysterectomy or ovarian surgery. Women who were still menstruating and those whose menopausal status was unknown were excluded. After exclusions were made, 436 ovarian cancer deaths were observed in the cohort. All the participants were assessed for general health, medical conditions, estrogen use (type, duration, dosage), medications and reproductive history. Among ever users, 52 percent had used Premarin (conjugated estrogen) and 36 percent did not remember the brand of hormone used. The questionnaire did not gather information on progestin use, nor was information on use of HRT available after 1982. However, before 1980, fewer than 5 percent of HRT prescriptions were for combined therapy. Women who used HRT (estrogen) were older, more likely to have an earlier menarche, older at menopause, previous use of oral contraceptives, lower body mass index and more formal education than nonusers. Follow-up was conducted every two years until 1988; since then, it has been conducted biannually through linkage with the National Death Index.

➤ Rodriguez C, Patel A, Calle E, Jacob E, and Thun M.

Estrogen replacement therapy and ovarian cancer mortality in a large prospective study of U.S. women. *Journal of the American Medical Association*, March 2001; 285:1460–1463. **Type:** Observational (cohort)

Focus: An examination of the association between postmenopausal estrogen use and ovarian cancer mortality.

Conclusions: Postmenopausal women who have used estrogens long-term (10 or more years) have an increased risk of ovarian cancer.

Findings:
- Postmenopausal women who had used HRT(estrogen) had an increased risk of ovarian cancer mortality (*rate ratio:* 1.23 for users/ 1.00 for nonusers).
- Risk was only slightly increased for former estrogen users (*rate ratio:* 1.16 for users/1.00 for nonusers).
- Duration and recency of use were predictors of risk.
- Women who had used HRT(estrogen) for ten years or more had a significant increased risk of ovarian cancer mortality (*rate ratio:* 2.20 for users/1.00 for nonusers).
- Risk of ovarian cancer mortality was only slightly increased for short duration (10 years or less) of use (*rate ratio:* 1.14 for users/1.00 for nonusers).

- Women who stopped estrogen had a decreased risk of ovarian cancer over time.

Researchers' Comments: "The impact of sequential or combined estrogen and progesterone therapy on ovarian cancer risk is unknown; additional large observational studies are needed to confirm our results and to examine whether effects are similar for unopposed estrogen use and estrogen used in combination with progesterone" (1464).

Participants and Methods: Data presented in this study is from the Cancer Prevention Study II, conducted from 1982 through 1996 in the United States and Puerto Rico. The female participants were postmenopausal women (211,581) who had completed a baseline questionnaire in 1982. These women had no history of cancer, hysterectomy or ovarian surgery at the time of enrollment. Women were excluded from the study for the following reasons: cancer, premenopausal status, unknown menopausal status, unknown age at menopause, incomplete data on estrogen use, injection of estrogen by cream or injection. The estrogen users in this study were more likely to be Caucasian, had more education, were leaner, had more tubal ligations and had fewer children than nonusers.

> ### Shu X, Brinton L, Gao Y, and Yuan J.

Population-based case-control study of ovarian cancer in Shanghai. **Cancer Research,** July 1989; 49:3670–3674. **Type:** Observational (case-control)

Focus: An investigation of the factors that contribute to the different ovarian cancer incidence rates among Chinese and American women.

Conclusions: Risk factors and medical factors are not the only determinants of different rates of ovarian cancer between Chinese and American women. Dietary factors may influence these differences. Hormone use, nulliparity, early menopause, family history of cancer, occupational exposure to paint and early menarche were associated with an increased risk of ovarian cancer. Oral contraceptives were not associated with a lower risk of ovarian cancer.

Findings:
- Women who used HRT (medroxyprogesterone) had an increased risk of ovarian cancer (**odds ratio:** 2.80 for users/1.00 for nonusers).
- Women who had used diethystilbestrol had an increased risk of ovarian cancer (**odds ratio:** 5.40 for users/1.00 for nonusers).
- Nulliparous women had a higher risk of ovarian cancer (**odds ratio:** 1.60).
- An early menopause, an early menarche and family history of cancer were associated with an increased risk of ovarian cancer.

- Sterilization and intrauterine contraceptives were associated with a reduced risk of ovarian cancer.
- Ovarian cancer risk was increased in women who had ovarian cysts or occupational exposure to paint.

Researchers' Comments: "Our study found use of medroxyprogesterone to be associated with a 2.8-fold increased risk of ovarian cancer, implying that progesterone might mechanistically relate to both ovarian cysts and ovarian cancer" (3674).

Participants and Methods: This study was conducted in a low-risk area for ovarian cancer, Shanghai China from 1984 to 1986. The cases were 229 women (18 to 70 years) diagnosed with ovarian cancer. These cases were matched with an population-based controls. The women were assessed for medical history, reproductive history, familial cancer history, demographics, lifestyle (personal habits, diet and occupation), and medication use (including hormones). Information was obtained through direct interviews and questionnaires.

➤ Weiss N, Lyon J, Krishnamurthy S, Dietert S, Liff J, and Daling J.

Noncontraceptive estrogen use and the occurrence of ovarian cancer. *Journal of the National Cancer Institute*, January 1982; 68:95–98.
Type: Observational (case-control)
Focus: An investigation of the use of HRT (estrogen) and its relationship to the occurrence of ovarian cancer in women.
Conclusions: HRT was associated with an increased risk of ovarian cancer, especially *endometrioid ovarian cancer.*
Findings:
- Women with epithelial ovarian tumors had used estrogen more than the control group.
- Women who had used HRT (estrogen) had an increased risk in all histologic types of epithelial ovarian cancer except the mucinous type.
- An elevated risk for endometrioid ovarian cancer was found in women who had received HRT, but this risk was not dose or duration related (**relative risk estimate:** 3.10 for users/1.00 for nonusers).
- Higher dosages of estrogen or longer duration of use were not associated with an increased risk of epithelial ovarian cancer.
- Seventeen women were diagnosed with endometrioid tumors and twelve of these women had used HRT (estrogen).

Researchers' Comments: "Several features of the association found here between the use of noncontraceptive estrogens and the incidence of ovarian endometrioid tumors suggest that the association may be real. The estimated risk to users relative to nonusers is high (about three times), and the diagnoses upon which this estimate is based appear accurate. In several areas of the United States, the reported incidence of endometrioid tumors increased during the early 1970's in parallel with the increasing use of noncontraceptive estrogens" (97).

Participants and Methods: The participants in this study were Caucasian women (50 to 74 years) who were residents of six counties in Utah and Washington and had been diagnosed with epithelial ovarian cancer from 1975 to 1979. The average interval from the time of diagnosis and the study interview was one year. Women (51 to 75 years) were recruited to be the control group using random telephone dialing and standard area sampling methods. Through interviews, the participants were assessed for general health, medical conditions, reproductive history, medications and estrogen use (dosage and type).

➤ Whittemore A, Harris R, Itnyre J, and the Collaborative Ovarian Cancer Group.

Characteristics relating to ovarian cancer risk: Collaborative analysis of 12 US case-control studies (Part I: Invasive epithelial ovarian cancers in white women). *American Journal of Epidemiology*, November 1992; 136:1184–1203. **Type:** Statistical (meta-analysis)

Focus: An examination of the risk factors for ovarian cancer based on the results from 12 U.S. studies.

Conclusions: Nulliparity is associated with an increased risk of ovarian cancer. Women who are infertile and engage in unprotected intercourse are at a higher risk for ovarian cancer. Pregnancy, breast feeding and oral contraceptive use are associated with a decreased risk of ovarian cancer. Age at first live birth, age at menarche, age at menopause and estrogen replacement do not appear to increase the risk of ovarian cancer.

Findings:

- Women who had used HRT generally had a decreased risk of ovarian cancer; however, population studies did find an increased risk in women who had used HRT for 10 to 15 years (**odds ratio:** 1.40 for users/1.00 for nonusers).
- No consistent trend of risk was associated with duration of estrogen replacement therapy: in hospital studies risk decreased with longer duration, with population studies risk increased with longer duration of use.

- Women, 40 years or younger who had hysterectomies, had a reduced risk of ovarian cancer if they had used estrogen replacement.
- The more pregnancies a woman had, the lower her risk of ovarian cancer and women who breast feed had a lower risk of ovarian cancer.
- Oral contraceptive use, tubal ligation and hysterectomy were associated with a lower risk of ovarian cancer.
- Women who had used fertility drugs had an increased risk of ovarian cancer.

Researchers' Comments: "We found no clear association between estrogen replacement therapy and risk of invasive ovarian cancer.... This lack of association contrasts with positive associations between estrogen therapy and cancers of the endometrium and possibly the breast, and it underscores the differences in the epidemiologies of these gynecologic malignancies" (1201).

Participants and Methods: This meta-analysis was based on data from 12 case-control studies conducted from 1956 to 1986. The participants were 2,197 Caucasian women with invasive epithelial ovarian cancer and 8,893 controls. Six of the studies analyzed were hospital studies with hospital controls and the other six studies were population studies with random digit dialing for neighborhood controls. Odds ratio estimates were adjusted for study, year of birth and reference age. Type and dosage of HRT were not defined in this analysis.

➤ Whittemore A (for the Collaborative Ovarian Cancer Group)

Personal characteristics relating to risk of invasive epithelial ovarian cancer in older women in the United States. *Cancer*, January 1993; 71: 558–565. **Type:** Statistical (meta-analysis)

Focus: An investigation of how the incidence of ovarian cancer varies among women based on age, reproductive characteristics and environmental factors.

Conclusions: No consistent risk factors were found associated with ovarian cancer in older women. Specific markers for and early detections of ovarian cancer are important in older women.

Findings:
- Ever use of HRT (estrogen alone) was not associated with an increased risk of ovarian cancer in hospital-based studies, but a slight risk was found in population-based studies **odds ratio:** 0.99 for users in hospital-based studies/1.10 in population-based studies/1.00 for nonusers).
- Nulliparous women had a higher risk of ovarian cancer.

- No clear trends in risk were identified for age at first live birth, parity and duration of oral contraceptive use or HRT and age at menopause.
- Years of *ovulation* were associated with an increased risk of ovarian cancer in younger women, but not older women.
- Among women less than 55 years, those with 35 or more years of ovulation had three times the risk of women with fewer than 25 years.
- Women who had breast-fed had a lower risk of ovarian cancer than those who did not breast feed.
- Women who had used oral contraceptive had a lower risk of ovarian cancer than women who had never used oral contraceptives, and risk decreased with increasing years of use.

Researchers' Comments: "The combined data showed no association between estrogen replacement therapy and ovarian cancer risk. This absence of association suggests that, if menopausal estrogen use affects risk, the effect is small. Additional data on risk among long-term users are needed to clarify this issue" (564).

Participants and Methods: The investigators examined age-related associations between ovarian cancer and reproductive/hormonal characters based on data from twelve case-control studies conducted in the United States from 1956 to 1986. The combined data detailed personal characteristics of 2197 Caucasian women with invasive epithelial ovarian cancer and 8893 controls.

6

Other Conditions

The studies that appear in this section include other conditions that are associated with or affected by HRT. Some of the studies in this section also deal with multiple conditions or general categories of disease, such as cancer. New topics include HRT and—colon cancer, cognitive functioning, lupus erythematosus, cancer risk factors, Alzheimer's disease, dementia, health characteristics of users, incontinence, menopausal symptoms, microalbuminuria, dry eye syndrome, exercise tolerance, neuromuscular functions, brain activation, dental health, urinary tract infections, adverse events, mortality, quality of life, obesity, mammography and breast density. Some of the studies are small, while others are large cohort or clinical trials. Two topics, cognitive functioning and colon cancer are of particular importance because more research is being conducted to explore the relationship between HRT and these conditions because of their impact on public health.

HRT, Cognitive Functioning and Alzheimer's Disease

Dementia and Alzheimer's disease are debilitating conditions for aging people and require expensive and extensive care. Alzheimer's is a progressive, degenerative disease of the brain and is the most common form of dementia. Alzheimer's disease is found in 2 to 3 percent of the general population, with 6 to 10 percent of people 65 years or older experiencing senile dementia related to Alzheimer's disease. The disease afflicts aging adults with most of its victims order than 65 years. With Alzheimer's, neural fibers become tangled and abnormal plaques are formed in the brain tissue. The

181

etiology of Alzheimer's disease is not known. Some casual theories include the loss of the enzyme choline acetyltransferase, uncontrolled ribonuclease (an enzyme that degrades RNA), the presence of prions (malformed proteins) and autoimmune agents such as antibodies that attack the brain tissue. Risk factors for the disease include a variation in the gene (E4 allele) that codes for the lipoprotein, apolipoprotein E. Alzheimer's tends to run in families and afflicts women more than men. Two types of the disease exist, early onset and late onset. Early onset is less common and is an inherited form of the disease. Symptoms of the Alzheimer's include inability to learn or recall new information, disorientation, and mental and physical deterioration over time. Those afflicted often lose the ability to communicate with or to recognize other people. Currently, no cure exists for the disease although certain drugs have been used to help manage it (e.g., tairine, donepezil).

Estrogen may provide protection against cognitive deterioration and brain disease by promoting the production of acetyltransferase, an important enzyme that makes neurons more responsive to nerve growth factors and connecting fibers. The evidence for a protective effect of estrogen on the brain is not conclusive, especially as a preventive treatment for Alzheimer's disease. The research is mixed with conflicting results. Some studies may be flawed due to a healthy user bias: women who receive HRT come from higher socioeconomic backgrounds, have a higher level of education, receive better and more consistent health care than those in the general population. Lengthy, well designed cohort and experimental studies are needed, and basic research should be conducted to understand the exact biological mechanism responsible for the disease.

(Love, 138–139; McCance & Huether, 444–445; http://www.nih.gov)

HRT and Colon Cancer

Colorectal cancer (cancer of the colon or rectum) is the third leading type of cancer in aging adults worldwide, the second most common cancer in Hispanic and black women, and the third most common cancer in Caucasian women. It is the second most frequent cause of cancer death in men and women. Between 1985 and 1995, colorectal cancer rates in the United States declined by 1.8 percent per year; since then, colorectal cancer rates have remained level. Mortality rates have also declined over the past 15 years by 1.7 percent per year. If diagnosed early, the prognosis is good and the 5-year survival rate is 62.1 percent. Colon cancer starts in the intestinal lining and grows to a size that causes bleeding and bowel obstruction. Symptoms include blood in the stools, changes in bowel habits, pain, and mass formation. Colon cancer arises from polyps, outgrowths of the lining of the colon that have become malignant. Polyps are asymptomatic and in most people present only a 1 percent chance of becoming malignant. However, some individuals carry a genetic predisposition (familial polyposis) to develop many precancerous malignant polyps that have a high probability of becoming cancerous. Risk of the disease increases after age 40 and rises sharply at ages 50 to 55. Risk factors for developing colon cancer identified in some, but not all studies include a family history, genetics, a history of ulcerative colitis, a diet high in fat (especially animal fat) and low in fiber, a history of other cancers, smoking, alcohol consumption and obesity. A reduced risk of colon cancer has been associated with a high fiber diet (from fruits and vegetables), physical exercise, calcium intake (e.g., low-fat dairy products), intake of vitamins E, folate and vitamin D, daily aspirin and HRT (estrogen). Preventative measure for colorectal cancer include colonoscopy with removal of polyps (beginning at age 50), sigmoidoscopy, barium enema and fecal occult blood testing.

HRT may be protective against the development of colon cancer, although the exact mechanism is not known. Estrogen and progesterone are thought to reduce the secretion of bile acids which can irritate the colon and increase the risk of cancer. Studies investigating the relationship between HRT and the development of colon cancer are still limited in number and duration. However, the existing studies show a protective effect of estrogen on the colon.

(Love, 138–139; McCance & Huether, 1257–1259; http://www.cancer.gov)

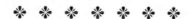

> **Adami H-O, Persson I, Hoover R, Schairer C, and Bergkvist L.**

Risk of cancer in women receiving hormone replacement therapy. *International Journal of Cancer*, November 1989; 44:833–839. **Type:** Observational (cohort)

Focus: An examination of the risk of cancer following HRT.

Conclusions: An increased risk of endometrial cancer and breast cancer was observed in women taking estrogens (e.g., conjugated estrogens or estradiol). Women receiving HRT had a lower risk of invasive cervical cancer; however, the researchers argue for cautious interpretation since these results may indicate more frequent pap tests and screening in these women than in the general population. Ovarian, pancreatic, colon and kidney cancer were not elevated in HRT users. The HRT users in this study showed a slightly lower risk of liver cancer. But there was an increased risk of malignant melanoma and lung cancer in women using HRT.

Findings:

- HRT users did not have an increased risk of kidney, liver, colon, ovarian or pancreatic cancer.
- Women who used HRT had an increased risk of breast cancer, lung cancer, endometrial cancer and malignant melanoma (**relative risk:** 1.11 for breast cancer, 1.26 for lung cancer, 1.78 for endometrial cancer, 1.45 for malignant melanoma).
- The researchers did not find a relationship between CNS (central nervous system) tumors and HRT.

Researchers' Comments: "This cohort had a higher number of smokers than in the general population" (838).

Participants and Methods: Women who had used HRT were identified through prescription forms from pharmacies in Uppsala health care region in Sweden. The recruitment for the study started in 1977, ended in 1980. The final cohort consisted of 77,147 prescription forms. The forms represented 23,244 women age 35 years or more. The mean age at entry was 54.5 years. The women were grouped according to the kinds of HRT used: potent estrogens (conjugated estrogens, 625 mg/d or 1.25 mg/d or estradiol), other estrogens (estriol compounds, 1–2 mg/d). In 1980, a subcohort was created in order to represent the women in the total cohort more accurately in terms of hormone exposure and potential confounding factors. The subcohort was chosen randomly and interviewed by questionnaires. These women were assessed for use of estrogen and use of progestagens. Follow-up of the subcohort occurred in 1982 and 1984. The researchers also wanted to know to what extent the cancer incidence in the general population might be confounded by a diverse distribution of risk factors for various malignant conditions. Therefore, for each woman in the subcohort, controls were selected randomly from the entire background population in the Uppsala health care region. The follow-up of the cohort continued to the end of 1984. The nation wide Registry of Causes of Death was used to determine dates of death and the National Cancer Registry was used to identify case of malignant diseases diagnosed in the study group.

▶ **Barrett-Connor E and Kritz-Silverstein D.**

Estrogen replacement therapy and cognitive function in older women. *Journal of the American Medical Association*, May 1993; 269:2637–2641. **Type:** Observational (cohort)

Focus: An examination of the effects of HRT on cognitive function in older women.

Conclusions: The evidence for a beneficial effect of HRT (estrogen) is not conclusive and is inconsistent. The data does not support the hypothesis that postmenopausal women receiving estrogen have better *cognitive* skills than nonusers.

Findings:

- Test scores of cognitive functions, adjusted for age and education, did not differ significantly by current, past or never use of estrogen.
- None of the 12 tests of cognitive function were consistently associated with current or past HRT (estrogen).
- Performance of 12 cognitive tests did not vary by duration or dosage of estrogen.
- Among 132 statistical comparisons, only five statistically significant differences were observed, less that the number expected by chance alone.

Researchers' Comments: "These divergent results may reflect the small numbers of subjects, limited number of psychometric tests used to evaluate cognitive function, or different estrogen regimens" (2640).

Participants and Methods: This study was based on data collected from a 1972 to 1974 in the Southern California upper-middle class community of Rancho Bernard. Participants were initially enrolled in a heart disease risk factor survey. Eighty percent of the surviving women from the original cohort, 800 women (65 to 95 years) provided the data for this study. The women were assessed for general health, medical conditions, reproductive history, medications and estrogen use. Estrogen use was evaluated at baseline (1972 to 1974) and at follow-up (1988 to 1991). Twelve tests of cognitive functioning were administered to the participants. Educational level did not vary by age and two-thirds of the women had completed some college.

➤ **Bergkvist L, Persson I, Adami H-O, and Schairer C.**

Risk factors for breast and endometrial cancer in a cohort of women treated with menopausal oestrogen. *International Journal of Epidemiology*, December 1988; 17:732–737. **Type:** Observational (cohort)

Focus: An investigation of the risk factors for breast cancer and endometrial cancer in women receiving HRT.

Conclusions: Women who have their ovaries surgically removed and later receive HRT have a lower risk of breast cancer.

Findings:

* The risk of diabetes and hypertension was not significant in women receiving HRT.
* Surgical menopause decreased the risk of breast cancer in women who received HRT.
* Type of menopause, education and prior breast biopsy were variables that affected a woman's risk of breast cancer.
* The prevalence of hysterectomy was important in determining a woman's risk of endometrial cancer.
* Women with more education were more inclined to receive HRT.

Researchers Comments: "Approximately 10 percent more of the women in the cohort than in the background population had undergone a hysterectomy, which has to be taken into account in the cohort analysis of endometrial cancer" (735).

Participants and Methods: The participants for this study were postmenopausal women recruited April 1977 to March 1980 through prescription forms from 120 pharmacies in Sweden. The final cohort involved 23,000 women who had received at least one prescription for HRT. These women were 35 years or older. The 735 women were randomly chosen from the cohort and designated as cases because they had used HRT. Controls, 1240 women, were obtained from a population register in the same area of Sweden. The controls were age-matched, two per each case. Women who responded to the questionnaires, formed the final cohort consisted of 735 cases and 952 controls. Cases and the controls were assessed through questionnaires about risk factors for breast and endometrial cancer, HRT and general medical health.

> ➤ **Boston Collaborative Drug Surveillance Program (Boston University Medical Center).**

Surgically confirmed gallbladder disease, venous thromboembolism and breast tumors in relation to postmenopausal estrogen therapy. *New England Journal of Medicine*, January 1974; 290:15–19. **Type:** Observational (case-control)

Focus: Data from many hospitals were examined to determine the relationship between HRT and the development of gallbladder disease, venous thromboembolism and breast tumors.

Conclusions: The risk of *gallbladder disease* is higher in women who receive HRT than in women who do not. HRT did not carry an elevated risk of venous thromboembolism or breast tumors.

Findings:

• The estimated incidence rate for gallbladder disease for healthy women who do not use HRT is 87 per 100,000 compared with 218 per 100,000 in women who use HRT.

• The risk of gallbladder disease increased in women who use HRT regardless of duration.

• Women who used HRT did not have an increased risk of venous thromboembolism.

Researchers' Comments: "The present findings show that the risk of gallbladder disease appears to be higher in postmenopausal women who use estrogens than in those who do not. The result is highly significant and chance is an unlikely explanation" (17).

Participants and Methods: The participants were drawn from 5,339 women interviewed and admitted to the medical and surgical wards of twenty-four hospitals in the Boston area between January and November 1972. The final study group, 774 cases, were postmenopausal women age 45 to 69 years. The cases were matched with a control group, 774 women, admitted to the hospital for acute illnesses, elective surgery or orthopedic treatment, were matched with the controls. Women who had a history of disease other than gallbladder disease, venous thromboembolism, breast tumors or hypertension were excluded from the study. The subjects were assessed for general health, medical conditions, reproductive status, lifestyle habits (cigarette, alcohol, coffee and tea consumption) and medicine use (including estrogen).

➤ **Brenner D, Kukull W, Stergachis A, van Belle G, Bowen J, McCormick W, Teri L, and Larson E.**

Postmenopausal estrogen replacement therapy and the risk of Alzheimer's disease: a population-based case-control study. *American Journal of Epidemiology*, August 1994; 140:262–267. **Type:** Observational (case-control)

Focus: An examination of the relationship between the development of Alzheimer's disease and the use of HRT.

Conclusions: HRT does not have a significant negative or positive effect on the risk of *Alzheimer's disease* in postmenopausal women. However, two groups of women who used HRT (oral estrogens & vaginal conjugated estrogens) had an increased risk of Alzheimer's disease.

Findings:

• Women who used HRT had a slight increase in the risk for Alzheimer's disease compared to women who never used HRT.

- Women who used HRT (all therapies considered) had a 10 percent greater risk of Alzheimer's disease than nonusers (**odds ratio:** 1.10 for users/1.00 for nonusers).
- Women who used vaginal estrogens had a 30 percent increased risk of Alzheimer's disease compared with nonusers.
- Women who had used vaginal estrogens and other oral estrogens had a higher risk of Alzheimer's than never users.

Researchers Comments: "The slightly varying odds ratios for different aspects of estrogen use are probably due to *random variation*" (265).

Participants and Methods: The participants were recruited from the Group Health Cooperative of Puget Sound, Seattle, Washington (health maintenance organization). These women were selected from a registry identifying individuals with symptoms of Alzheimer's disease. All participants were assessed for HRT use and medical history; given physical and neurological examinations. Eligible cases were women enrolled in the Alzheimer's Disease Patient Registry between April 1987 and February 1992. The final study group consisted of 107 cases and 180 controls The control group was selected from the same Group Health Cooperative of Puget Sound. The cases and controls were matched for age and other characteristics. The controls had no indication of dementia on the basis of psychometric and clinical evaluation.

➤ **Byrd B, Burch J, and Vaughn W.**

The impact of long-term estrogen support after hysterectomy. *The Annals of Surgery*, May 1977; 185:574–580. **Type:** Observational (cohort)

Focus: An investigation of the effects of long term estrogen use in women who had undergone hysterectomies.

Conclusions: Long term HRT by women who have had hysterectomies is favorable. The overall mortality from all diseases was less in the women who had used HRT. The researchers found a steady decline in cancer cases in all age groups after 10 years of estrogen therapy. However, the risk of breast cancer increased in women who had used HRT for ten years or less.

Findings:
- Women who used HRT had lower *mortality* from all causes.
- Women who had used HRT showed less evidence of osteoporosis than women who did not use HRT.
- An increased breast cancer risk was found in women who used HRT for at least 10 years.
- Nulliparous women may be at a higher risk of cancer during the first 10 years of HRT.

• Women who have a late menopause and are nulliparous have an increased risk of breast cancer.

Researchers' Comments: " Since women who have a late menopause and who are nulliparous have an increased risk for breast cancer, special considerations must be given to the initiation of estrogen therapy after age 55. ... [T]hese factors identify a group who are at special risk to develop breast cancer and the role of estrogen in these individuals is as yet poorly established" (578).

Participants and Methods: The subjects were 1016 Caucasian women from Tennessee (22–78 years) who had undergone hysterectomies, and were given conjugated estrogen (1.25 mg/day). This group was followed by contact and questionnaires. The study group consisted of patients of one author of this study. These women were given estrogen for three or more years. Information that appeared in this article was the result of the second or third follow-up since 1970. The group was assessed for nulliparity, ovarian status, age at birth of first child and health status.

▶ **Calle E, Miracle-McMahill H, Thun M, and Heath C.**

Estrogen replacement therapy and risk of fatal colon cancer in a prospective cohort of postmenopausal women. *Journal of the National Cancer Institute*, April 1995; 87:517–523. **Type:** Observational (Cohort)

Focus: An investigation of the relationship between fatal colon cancer and HRT use among postmenopausal women.

Conclusions: Current users and long-term users of HRT have a decreased risk of fatal colon cancer.

Findings:
• Women who used HRT (estrogen alone) had a decreased risk of fatal colon cancer (**relative risk:** 0.71 for users/1.00 for nonusers).
• Current users of estrogen had the lowest risk of fatal colon cancer (**relative risk:** 0.55 for users/1.00 for nonusers).
• The risk of fatal colon cancer decreased the longer a woman used HRT.
• Former users of estrogen had a reduced risk of fatal colon cancer (**relative risk:** 0.62 for users within 10 years/0.85 for users of 11 years or more/1.00 for nonusers).

Researchers' Comments: "Women who use postmenopausal estrogens differ from nonusers with regard to a number of possible confounding factors that could influence health and survival. Estrogen users tend to be better educated, to be white, to be leaner, to exercise more often, to be nonsmokers, and to use preventive health services more often than nonusers.... Women who receive estrogens may have more intensive medical surveillance and may thus be diagnosed earlier, when survival from colon cancer is better. While we cannot rule out the possibility that surveillance bias might have affected our results, the reduction in risk associated with estrogen use appears too large to be explained fully by such a bias" (520).

Participants and Methods: Women in this study were selected from the 676,526 female (45 to 70 years) participants in the Cancer Prevention Study II. This study of mortality involved approximately 1.2 million American men and women initiated by the American Cancer Society in 1982. Participants were enrolled by the American Cancer Society volunteers throughout the United States. These volunteers made inquires in 1984, 1986 and 1988 to determine if enrollees were alive or deceased, and recorded date and place of deaths. The female participants were assessed through questionnaires for demographic characteristics, environmental exposures, lifestyle, personal and family history of cancer, medical conditions, estrogen use, reproductive history and medications. After seven years of follow-up, 897 eligible cases of fatal colon cancer were observed among 422,373 postmenopausal women who were cancer free upon entering the study.

➤ **Col N, Pauker S, Goldberg R, Eckman M, Orr R, Ross E, and Wong J.**

Individualizing therapy to prevent long-term consequences of estrogen deficiency in postmenopausal women. *Archives of Internal Medicine*, July 1999; 159:1458–1466. **Type:** Statistical

Focus: An examination of the risks and benefits of different therapies to help women and health care providers make decisions regarding treatment.

Conclusions: Each woman should be individually assessed for her risk for hip fracture, coronary heart disease and breast cancer to decide the best therapy. Any of the therapies are justified if they provide a gain in life expectancy of at least six months; however, the benefit of each therapy depends upon a woman's risk factors. Based on life expectancy, the benefits of treatment for osteoporosis are small compared with the treatment impact on heart disease and breast cancer.

Findings:
- Women who have a low risk of coronary heart disease, breast cancer and hip fracture do not benefit significantly from any treatment.
- Women who benefit from HRT (raloxifene) are those with a low risk of coronary heart disease but at high risk of breast cancer.

- Women who benefit from HRT (combined therapy) are those at high risk for coronary heart disease or at average risk for coronary heart disease, breast cancer and hip fracture.
- HRT (raloxifene, estrogen alone, combined therapy) and *alendronate* reduce the risk of hip fractures (**relative risk:** 0.58 for raloxifene/0.57 for estrogen and combined therapy/ 0.54 for alendronate).
- Women with average risks of coronary heart disease, breast cancer and hip fracture benefit from HRT (raloxifene) if it lowers their risk of breast cancer by at least 66 percent.
- An increased risk of breast cancer of 47 percent exists with HRT (estrogen + progestin).

Researchers' Comments: "We could not completely explore the impact of quality of life and personal preferences in our analysis. Individuals vary in their perceptions and valuations of outcomes affected by these therapies, and we lack accurate methods to measure these preferences on an individual basis. Because the risk of HRT includes breast cancer which many women fear more than CHD or hip fractures, any gains in life expectancy from HRT must be balanced against an individual's desire to avoid breast cancer.... Raloxifene and alendronate were approved for the primary prevention of osteoporosis based on less than 3 years of clinical trial experience. For some, this may be an insufficient duration to be confident of the long-term impact of these therapies on fracture risk, breast cancer or the clinical end points" (1463).

Participants and Methods: In this statistical study the researchers employed a decision model to analyze the impact of different treatment protocols (HRT—combined therapy, raloxifene and alendronate) on hip fractures, coronary heart disease, breast cancer and life expectancy in postmenopausal women with different risk factors. Other statistical models (regression models) were employed to relate individual risks factors to future disease risks and the impact of treatment of these. Low risk was defined as the absence of any risk factors; high risk was associated with the two or more known risk factors for that disease. Low risk for hip fracture was defined as the absence of any risk factors among women whose weight had increased more than 20 percent since age twenty-five. Low risk factor for coronary heart disease was defined as the absence of any risk factors and having a total HDL/total cholesterol ratio of less than 2.8 and a systolic blood pressure less than 125 mm hg. Low risk for breast cancer was defined as having no first-degree relatives with breast cancer, having no previous breast biopsies and being less than 25 years of age at first live birth. High risk of breast cancer was defined as having two or more first-degree relatives with breast cancer.

➤ **Conner E and Kritz-Silverstein D.**

Estrogen replacement therapy and cognitive function in older women. *Journal of the American Medical Association*, May 1993; 269:2637–2641. **Type:** Observational (cohort)

Focus: An investigation of the role estrogen plays in the mental functioning of older women.

Conclusions: HRT did not preserves mental functioning in older women. However, on one test women who had used estrogen in the past performed better than non-users or estrogen long-term users. A few other tests showed minor differences.

Findings:

- Current users of HRT did not differ significantly from nonusers on any cognitive test.
- No significant differences in mental abilities with duration or dose of estrogen except for a test of short-term recall where short-term users of HRT had the best results.
- Women who had used HRT for less than 2 years had better scores on short-term recall tests than those women who had used HRT for 3–10 years.
- Based on duration of use, on the test of category fluency the women who had used estrogen for a long duration scored better than non-users and short-term users.

Researchers' Comments: "In spite of the multiple comparisons in which one might have expected some significant benefit by chance alone, only five statistically significant differences independent of age and education were found among 132 statistical comparisons; the differences were not consistent for any specific test of cognitive function and in three instances women who were treated in the past with estrogen scored better than women currently receiving treatment" (2640).

Participants and Methods: The study involved 800 women, 65 to 95 years old recruited from Rancho Bernardo, a community in Southern California. These women were originally part of a heart disease risk factor survey conducted from 1972 to 1974. The researchers compared performance on 12 items from eight standard tests of cognitive function. The women were asked about estrogen use and requestioned during follow-up. Most of the women receiving HRT, used Premarin (unopposed conjugated estrogen). Between 1988 and 1991, 80 percent of the surviving women participated in a follow-up clinic which included tests of mental functioning.

➤ **Davies G, Hustler W, Lu Y, Ploufee L,
and Lakshmanan M.**

Adverse events reported by postmenopausal women in controlled trials with raloxifene. *Obstetrics and Gynecology*, April 1999; 93:558–
565. **Type:** Statistical (meta-analysis)

Focus: An assessment of the incidence of adverse events in postmenopausal women receiving raloxifene compared with other forms of
HRT and placebo.

Conclusions: Raloxifene treated women had more hot flashes than
HRT groups (estrogen alone or combined therapy) but less breast pain or
vaginal bleeding.

Findings:
• Raloxifene treated women did not experience more adverse events
  compared with women receiving other forms of HRT.
• Women who received raloxifene did not have more vaginal bleeding
  than the placebo groups.
• HRT groups experienced 89 percent bleeding in the cyclic combined
  therapy group and 64 percent in the continuous combined therapy
  group.
• Raloxifene treated women had more hot flashes than women receiving
  other forms of HRT.
• Leg cramps were reported more often in raloxifene treated women
  than in placebo controlled groups.
• Raloxifene treated women and placebo treated women experienced
  less breast pain than the HRT (estrogen and combined therapy)
  groups that reported more breast pain.

Researchers' Comments: "A very rare but significant adverse event
associated with postmenopausal hormone therapy is an approximately
threefold increase in the incidence of venous thromboembolism. A similar risk was observed for raloxifene in an ongoing, large-scale osteoporosis
treatment trial of over 7000 postmenopausal women ... and raloxifene is
contraindicated in women with current or previous venous thromboembolic events" (564).

Participants and Methods: The researchers analyzed data from
eight, randomized clinical trials (six to thirty months duration) involving
2789 postmenopausal women. Similar treatment groups were pooled and
databases were created. The data included information about adverse effects
in placebo groups, estrogen alone groups and combined therapy groups.
In the trials analyzed, the women received one of these treatments: raloxifene (60 mg/d), conjugated estrogen alone (0.625 mg/d), cyclic combined

therapy (conjugated equine estrogen, 0.625 mg/d plus medroxyprogesterone acetate, 5 mg/d), or conjugated equine estrogen (0.625 mg/d plus norgestrel, 0.15 mg/d), continuous combined therapy (conjugated equine estrogen, 0.625 mg/d plus medroxyprogesterone acetate, 2.5 mg/d) or placebo. The progestin was taken on cycle days 7–28 in cyclic HRT regimens. All the participants were assessed for general health, medical conditions, estrogen use, reproductive history and medications. Women were excluded if they had a history of estrogen-dependent cancers, cancer within the previous five years, treatment with androgens or estrogen (within six months of enrollment except one trial), treated for osteoporosis or high cholesterol, showed abnormal kidney or liver function, or had extreme vasomotor symptoms (e.g., hot flashes). Participants were interviewed to obtain information regarding adverse events.

➤ Derby C, Hume A, McPhillips J, Barbour M, and Carleton R.

Prior and current health characteristics of postmenopausal estrogen replacement therapy users compared with nonusers. *The American Journal of Obstetrics and Gynecology*, August 1995; 173:544–550. **Type:** Observational (cohort)

Focus: An investigation whether the selection of healthy women for postmenopausal estrogen therapy confounds studies of estrogen use and cardiovascular disease risk.

Conclusions: Selection of healthy women for HRT studies does not completely explain the reduction of cardiovascular risk that have been observed. Postmenopausal users appear to have more healthy lifestyles than do nonusers in terms of smoking, exercise and medical monitoring (e.g., cholesterol tests). Cardiovascular benefits of estrogen replacement therapy may be overestimated in observational studies. More healthy lifestyles among women selected for HRT would tend to inflate the apparent benefits of treatment for cardiovascular disease.

Findings:
- Estrogen users were less likely to be smokers and more likely to exercise regularly.
- Estrogen users were more likely to have their cholesterol checked regularly.
- HDL cholesterol was significantly higher in HRT users.
- More estrogen users reported vigorous exercise at least once per week and alcohol consumption in the past 24 hours.

Researchers' Comments: "The frequency of estrogen use was low in the analysis population and the majority of women using estrogen were those with surgical menopause. This reflects the low prevalence of estrogen use in these communities throughout the study period, particularly among women with natural menopause. To the extent that differences between estrogen users and nonusers vary by type of menopause, studies in which the majority of estrogen users are women with surgical menopause may be biased" (549).

Participants and Methods: This study compared postmenopausal women who used estrogen with postmenopausal women who did not use estrogen. The analysis included characteristics of the women before and during the time of estrogen use. The data was obtained from two independent cohorts as part of the evaluation component of the Pawtucket Heart Health Program. This program was created to test whether cardiovascular morbidity and mortality could be reduced through community risk factor intervention. Data were gathered from a baseline (1981–1984) and followed-up (1990–1992) with health surveys of two cohorts randomly selected from some communities in southeastern New England. The data analyzed included the following: cigarette smoking status, cholesterol level measured in the past year, alcohol consumption in the past 24 hours, dietary intake of fat and salt, ages and income, body mass index and the presence of regular exercise.

> **Ettinger B, Friedman G, Bush T, and Quesenberry C.**

Reduced mortality associated with long-term postmenopausal estrogen therapy. ***Obstetrics and Gynecology***, January 1996; 87:6-12. **Type:** Observational (case control)

Focus: An investigation of all-cause and specific cause mortality rates in women who had used long-term postmenopausal estrogen replacement therapy.

Conclusions: Long-term HRT is associated with lower all-cause mortality and provides a reduction in cardiovascular disease. Women who used estrogen replacement therapy also had a lower risk of lung cancer mortality even if they smoked. However, the researchers found that estrogen users had a higher risk of death from breast cancer than nonusers.

Findings:

• The relative risk of death from all causes associated with 25 or more years of estrogen use was lower than shorter duration of its use.
• The relative risk of death was lowest among those women using the lowest dosage of estrogen.

- The higher doses of estrogen were not associated with a higher risk of mortality.
- A reduction in mortality from coronary heart disease and from cardiovascular disease was found among estrogen users.
- HRT was associated with a 30 percent increased risk of breast cancer mortality, especially long term users.

Researchers Comments: "Use of estrogen in this cohort was almost entirely unopposed by progestin, which thereby limits extrapolation of our results to the many women who now use combined HRT" (11).

Participants and Methods: In 1980, using computer pharmacy records, researchers identified 110 women born from 1900 to 1915 who had used estrogen during the years 1969–1973. Two groups were selected. One group included women who had used postmenopausal estrogen for at least five years, and the other group was of age-matched women who had not used estrogen for less than one year. The women were chosen from a large health maintenance organization and their follow-up consisted of analysis of individual medical records and computer data bases. Women who had heart problems, stroke or cancer were excluded from the study. The final study group was composed of 232 estrogen users and 222 nonusers. In 1993 the researchers found that most of the women in the original cohort were still health plan members; their mean age was 77 years and the mean duration of estrogen use was 17 years or more.

➤ **Fantl J, Bump R, Robinson D, McClish D, Wyman J, and the Continence Program for Women Research Group.**

Efficacy of estrogen supplementation in the treatment of urinary incontinence. *Obstetrics and Gynecology*, November 1996; 88:745–749.
Type: Experimental (clinical trial)

Focus: An examination the effectiveness of HRT in treating incontinence in postmenopausal women with low levels of estrogen.

Conclusions: Women who received HRT did not report an improvement in *urinary incontinence*. Estrogen was no more effective than the placebo used in this clinical trial.

Findings:
- Outcome measurements for the HRT group and the control group were the same.
- No difference existed between the HRT group and control group reports of quality of life issues.

- Women who used HRT did not show improvement with urinary incontinence.

Researchers' Comments: "The use of ... progestin therapy could account for some of the observed lack of response, as there is some evidence that progesterone may have the opposite effect of estrogens in the lower urinary tract" (748).

Participants and Methods: This randomized clinical trial (placebo-controlled/double blind) recruited participants from the Medical College of Virginia, Virginia Commonwealth University and Bowman Gray School of Medicine, Wake Forest University. The study involved 833 postmenopausal women (45 years), who had involuntary loss of urine at least once a week. The outcome for the study was a measurement of the number of incontinent episodes per week as recorded by patients. The patients were also assessed for quantity of urine loss, voluntary daytime urination, nighttime urination and quality of life. A health survey and the Center for Epidemiological Studies Depression Scale were used to assess quality of life. Patients were also asked to rate their perception of improvement using five categories of responses (worse or better). The women were randomized to receive either a placebo or HRT. Subjects in the treatment group received conjugated equine estrogen (0.625mg/d) for 30 days and medroxyprogesterone (10mg) for 10 days of each cycle. Women in the control group received placebo tablets in a cyclic regimen. All data collected at baseline were gathered after this three-month study.

➤ **Genant H, Lucas J, Weiss S, Akin M, Emkey R, McNaney-Flint H, Downs R, Watts N, Mortola J, Yang H, Banav N, Brennan J, and Nolan J.**

Low-dose esterified estrogen therapy: effects on bone, plasma estradiol concentrations, endometrium, and lipid levels. *Archives of Internal Medicine,* December 1997; 157:2609–2615. **Type:** Experimental (clinical trial)

Focus: An investigation of the effect of various dosages of *esterified estrogen* on bone loss, the endometrium, lipid levels and plasma estradiol concentrations in postmenopausal women.

Conclusions: Women who received esterified estrogens (unopposed) had positive changes in bone mass and lipid profiles. Esterified estrogen (0.3 mg/d) was effective at increasing bone mass without inducing endometrial hyperplasia. However, higher doses of esterified estrogen resulted in adverse endometrial conditions in some women.

Findings:
- Endometrial hyperplasia was a major cause of women dropping out of

the study and discontinuing estrogen therapy; particularly in those groups that received higher dosages of esterified estrogen (0.625 and 1.25 mg/d).

- All dosages of esterified estrogens resulted in increased bone mineral density, especially in the women receiving 1.25 mg/d.
- More vaginal bleeding occurred in women who received 0.625 or 1.25 mg/d esterified estrogens than in the placebo or 0.3 mg/d groups.
- LDL cholesterol was decreased and HDL cholesterol was increased in all women who received esterified estrogens; the highest increase in HDL cholesterol was in the group receiving 0.625mg/d.
- Adverse reactions that resulted in women stopping the HRT were headaches and vaginal bleeding which increased with higher dosages.

Researchers' Comments: "The bone mineral density results reported herein may not apply to conjugated equine estrogens, which contain different amounts and ratios of estrone, equilin, and other estrogenic constituents" (2614).

Participants and Methods: This two year, randomized clinical trial (double blind) involving 218 postmenopausal women, was initiated in twenty-nine investigation centers throughout the United States. The women were assessed at baseline and at six month intervals for the following: bone mineral density (dual X-ray absorptiometry), lipid profile, endometrial status (biopsy) and blood estradiol levels. General health was also monitored, and none of the women were smokers or previous users of HRT. Women who had received medication that would affect bone mineral metabolism were excluded from the study. The women were randomly assigned to one of four treatment protocols: placebo, esterified estrogen (0.3 mg/d), esterified estrogen (0.625 mg/d) or esterified estrogen (1.25 mg/d). The women were also told to take 1000 mg/d of calcium (OsCal or Citracal) in divided doses per day.

▶ **Greendale G, Reboussin B, Hogan P, Barnabei V, Shumaker S, Johnson S, and Barrett-Connor E (for the PEPI Trial Investigators).**

Symptom relief and side effects of postmenopausal hormones: results from the postmenopausal estrogen/progestin intervention trial. *Obstetrics and Gynecology*, December 1998; 92:982–988. **Type:** Experimental (clinical trial)

Focus: An assessment of the effectiveness of HRT to relieve menopausal symptoms and an evaluation of the side-effects of HRT

Conclusions: HRT relieves vasomotor symptoms. Combined therapy (estrogen + progestin) causes breast discomfort. HRT does not affect psychological symptoms such as anxiety or cognitive functioning.

Findings:

• Combined therapy (estrogen + progestin) was not better than estrogen alone in treating vasomotor symptoms such as hot flashes.

• Women who received HRT did not experience weight gain.

• Women who received combined therapy, either estrogen + progestin or estrogen + progesterone had fewer muscular-skeletal symptoms (e.g., joint pain).

• Anxiety, cognitive functioning and affective symptoms did not vary among the treatment groups.

Researchers' Comments: "Many of the known side effects of HRT have not been evaluated in placebo-controlled clinical trials" (983).

Participants and Methods: The three-year PEPI trial (randomized/double blind) was initiated in 1989 and involved 875 postmenopausal women (45 to 64 years) at seven clinical centers in the United States. The women were assessed for general health, medical conditions, lifestyle (exercise, alcohol and cigarette consumption) reproductive history, medications and estrogen use. Symptoms were evaluated using a checklist at baseline, 12 months and at 36 months. Participants were assigned to one of the following treatment groups: placebo, conjugated equine estrogen, conjugated equine estrogens plus cyclical medroxyprogesterone acetate, or conjugated equine estrogen plus micronized progesterone.

➤ **Grodstein F, Stampfer M, Goldhaber S, Manson J, Colditz G, Speizer F, Willett W, and Hennekens C.**

Prospective study of exogenous hormones and risk of pulmonary embolism in women. *Lancet*, October 1996; 348:983–987. **Type:** Observational (cohort)

Focus: An investigation of the relationship between the use HRT and pulmonary embolism.

Conclusions: Women who are current users of HRT have an increased risk of *pulmonary embolism.*

Oral contraceptives were also associated with an increased risk of pulmonary embolism.

Findings:

• Pulmonary embolism was uncommon in this study group but an increased risk was associated with current estrogen use (***relative risk:*** 2.10 for users/1.00 for nonusers).

- Past users of HRT had only a slight increase in risk of pulmonary embolism (*relative risk:* 1.30 for past users/1.00 for users).
- Duration of estrogen use did not affect the risk of pulmonary embolism: current users of HRT (five or more years) had an increased risk of primary pulmonary embolism with a *relative risk* of 1.90; however, current users of estrogen (five years or less) had a higher *relative risk* of 2.60.
- The dosage of estrogen did not significantly affect the risk of pulmonary embolism (*relative risk:* 1.90 in women receiving of estrogen, 0.3 mg/d; 1.50 in women receiving estrogen 0.625 mg/d and 1.40 in women receiving estrogen 1.25 mg or more daily).
- Women who smoked cigarettes and used HRT did not have a higher risk of pulmonary embolism than women who used HRT but did not smoke.

Researchers' Comments: "In this large prospective study, women currently using postmenopausal hormones had a significantly increased risk of primary pulmonary embolism" (985).

Participants and Methods: The data for this study was derived from the Nurses' Health Study, a prospective study which involved 112,593 female nurses (30–55 years) from 1976 to 1992 living in eleven states. The women were followed up every two years with questionnaires. The women were assessed form general health, medical conditions, medications used, cardiovascular risk factors, reproductive history and HRT (type and duration). The dosage of HRT was included beginning in 1980. During the follow-up time of this study, most of the postmenopausal women used estrogen alone without progestin. Women were excluded from the study if they had a previous history of pulmonary embolism, cancer (except nonmelanoma skin cancer), cardiovascular conditions, stroke or incomplete information about estrogen usage.

➤ Grodstein F, Stampher M, Colditz G, Willett W, Manson J, Joffe M, Rosner B, Fuchs C, Hankinson S, Hunter D, Hennekens C, and Speizer F.

Postmenopausal hormone therapy and mortality. *The New England Journal of Medicine*, June 1997; 336:1769–1775. **Type:** Observational (cohort)

Conclusions: Women who used HRT generally had a lower mortality, but this lowered mortality stopped after five years of discontinued therapy. Women who received HRT had a reduced mortality especially from cardiovascular disease; however, women who initially had a lower risk of heart disease did not benefit substantially from HRT. A 43 percent increased risk of breast cancer was observed in women who used HRT after 10 years of use. Because of this increased breast cancer risk, there was no benefit from hormones with increasing duration of use.

Findings:

- Current hormone use did not have an increase in mortality and generally had a lower mortality for all causes than nonusers (*relative risk:* 0.63 for users/1.00 for never users).
- Based on duration of use, HRT users had increased mortality because of an increase in breast cancer (*relative risk:* 1.16 for users for five or more years/1.00 for never users).
- Past users of HRT had an increased mortality for some conditions (*relative risk:* 1.04 for all cancers; 1.07 for stroke).
- Adjustments for diet, alcohol consumption, vitamin or aspirin use and exercise did not affect the relative risk.
- 3637 deaths occurred between 1976 and 1994 among postmenopausal women in the study: 461 died of coronary heart disease, 167 died of stroke and 1985 died of cancer (425 were of breast cancer).

Researchers' Comments: "We observed no increasing benefit of hormones with increasing duration of use; in contrast, the apparent benefits were attenuated after 10 or more years of current hormone use. Whereas lower rates of cardiovascular mortality were maintained for long-term users, the risk of breast cancer mortality in this population was elevated by 43 percent after 10 years of taking hormones. Thus, with additional years of use, expected mortality advantages were, in part, offset by the risk of breast cancer; this was true even for the oldest women in the cohort (those 60 to 73 years of age)" (1773).

Participants and Methods: The Nurses' Health Study began in 1976 with data from mailed questionnaires of 121,700 women (30–55 years). The women were assessed for general medical history, menopausal status, cardiovascular and cancer risk factors, and hormone use. For each case subject, ten controls were chosen at random from among women alive at the time of the case subjects' death or at the time of the diagnosis of the disease leading to death. Biennial follow-up questionnaires were used to update information on risk factors and newly diagnosed illnesses. Women were excluded from the study if they had a history of cardiovascular disease or cancer (except nonmelanoma skin cancer).

➤ Hammond C, Jelovsek F, Lee K, Creasman W, and Parker R.

Effects of long-term estrogen replacement therapy: II Neoplasia. *American Journal of Obstetrics and Gynecology*, March 1979; 133:537–546. **Type:** Observational (cohort)

Focus: The second part of a study of two groups of women assessing the relationship of long-term HRT and neoplasia.

Conclusions: Women who used HRT (conjugated estrogen) had an increased incidence of endometrial cancer. Long-term use of HRT did not result in a higher than an expected incidence of other cancers.

Findings:

- HRT users who received estrogen alone had increased risk for endometrial cancer (**risk ratio:** 9.30 for white women/1.10 for nonusers).
- The **risk ratio** for all cancer sites was 1.92 for white estrogen users and 1.03 for nonwhite estrogen users.
- The addition of progesterone (combined therapy) provided significant protection against the development of endometrial cancer.
- The addition of progestin to estrogen therapy did not reduce the benefit of estrogen treatment on metabolism.
- No significant increased risk of breast cancer was found in long-term users of HRT.

Researchers' Comments: "Of concern was the finding that all 11 of the women with adenocarcinoma of the endometrium received estrogen by cyclic administration (usually 25 days per month). Thus, the thesis that cyclic estrogen therapy may be protective against this may not be warranted" (545).

Participants and Methods: The participants were two groups of women identified through Duke University Medical Center, Durham, North Carolina. The women were selected because of a diagnosis related to a hypoestrogenic condition. These women had been observed at the medical center for at least five years (initially around 1974). The medical charts of the women were used to gather information about each patient's health status, medications and general medical history. The two groups were then selected on the basis of those receiving estrogen and those who were nonusers. There were 301 women receiving HRT, mostly conjugated estrogen (Premarin); there were 309 women who did not receive HRT. The two groups were then analyzed to determine the incidence rates of neoplasms.

> **Haskell S, Richardson E, and Horwitz R.**

The effect of estrogen replacement therapy on cognitive function in women: A critical review of the literature. *Journal of Clinical Epidemiology*, November 1997; 50:1249–1264. **Type:** Qualitative Analysis

Focus: An examination of the effects of HRT (estrogen) on cognitive function found in clinical trials.

Conclusions: Some observational studies support the beneficial effects of estrogen on cognitive functioning; however, the data from the clinical trials do not support the conclusion that estrogen improves cognitive functioning in post-menopausal women or women with Alzheimer's disease.

Findings:

- A comparison of the studies, showed major differences (heterogeneity) between the subjects, treatments and tests used to assess changes in cognitive functioning.
- Variability existed between the studies in the kinds of measurements used to determine cognitive functioning.
- Clinical trials that claimed benefit from estrogen therapy did not control for confounding variables such as depression and *vasomotor symptoms*.
- Five of the nine observational studies found some association between estrogen use and cognitive functioning.
- Three of the ten randomized trials found significant improvement in memory in participants receiving estrogen and two showed improvement in memory.

Researchers' Comments: "Perhaps the most striking observation in our review of these 19 studies is the extreme heterogeneity in subjects, treatments and tests used to assess change in cognitive function. Treatment regimens showed just as much heterogeneity as baseline characteristics of the women. In one study, women received a large dose of estradiol (4 mg) daily, whereas another study chose to use as little as 0.5 mg of estradiol with a progesterone. But clearly, the most remarkable and disappointing aspect of these studies was their failure to define suitably valid and reliable measures of outcome" (1262).

Participants and Methods: Nineteen studies were analyzed using MEDLINE to search publications between 1970 and 1996: ten randomized controlled tails, two uncontrolled trials, one cross-sectional study, four case-control studies and one prospective cohort study. Each study was examined for baseline characteristics of the subject and eligibility criteria, duration of the follow-up and method of treatment. The psychological tests used in each study were examined for validity and reliability.

➤ Hemminki E and McPherson K.

Impact of postmenopausal hormone therapy on cardiovascular events and cancer, pooled data from clinical trials. *British Medical Journal*, July 1997; 315:149–153. **Type:** Statistical (meta-analysis)

Focus: An examination of the incidence of cardiovascular diseases and cancer from clinical trials.

Conclusions: HRT does not prevent cardiovascular disease or related conditions.

Findings:

- Women who received HRT had an increased risk of thromboembolisms (*odds ratio:* 2.89 for users/1.00 for nonusers).
- Women who received HRT had an increased risk of cardiovascular conditions (*odds ratio:* 1.39 for users/1.00 for nonusers).
- Women who used HRT did not have an increased risk of cancer.
- Women who did not receive HRT had fewer cardiovascular problems and thromboembolic conditions.

Researchers' Comments: "The result of these pooled (mostly) randomized data do not support the notion that postmenopausal hormone therapy prevents cardiovascular events" (153).

Participants and Methods: The studies analyzed were obtained through Medline database and bibliographies. The researches pooled the data to determine the incidence of cardiovascular disease and cancer in HRT users. Twenty-two trials were examined with 4124 participating women. The women in these trial either received some form of estrogen alone or combined therapy (estrogen + progestin or progesterone). In each group, the number of women with cardiovascular or cancerous conditions were summed and divided by the number of women originally assigned to the group. Trials with three months or more of treatment were included.

➤ Henderson B, Paganini-Hill A, and Ross R.

Decreased mortality in users of estrogen replacement therapy. *Archives of Internal Medicine*, January 1991; 151:75–78. **Type:** Observational (cohort)

Focus: An investigation of the relationship of HRT and mortality.

Conclusions: Current users of HRT have a low death rate in the elderly population. Mortality decreased with increasing duration of HRT. The reduced mortality was due to fewer deaths from *arteriosclerosis*.

Findings:

- HRT users had a reduced mortality form cancer.

- Women who had used HRT for more than 15 years had a reduced mortality.
- Mortality from all remaining causes combined was the same in estrogen users and nonusers.
- The mortality for those women who had used conjugated estrogens at a dosage of 0.625 mg/d or less was lower than that for women whose dosage was 1.25 mg/d or greater.
- Estrogen users had a reduced rate of mortality from arteriosclerotic disease and *cerebrovascular disease*.

Researchers' Comments: One possible explanation for these findings is that estrogen users may have less extensive disease at diagnosis than nonusers owing to increased medical surveillance or to better health awareness among women using medications.... Despite the substantial overall mortality benefit afforded estrogen users, if the decision is to begin therapy, it is imperative that both physician and patient place high priority on surveillance of unexplained uterine bleeding and breast lumps" (78).

Participants and Methods: In 1981 a prospective study of 8881 postmenopausal residents in a retirement community in Southern California was initiated. A health questionnaire was mailed to the residents of Leisure World, Laguna Hills. New residents who moved into the community after 1981 were mailed the questionnaire in June 1982, June 1983 and October 1985. The median age at the time of mailing was 73 years. The women were questioned about current health and prior conditions, height and weight, smoking and alcohol consumption, exercise, reproductive history and hormone use. The most commonly used HRT was conjugated estrogen (Premarin). The cohort was followed-up for deaths and two follow-up mailings occurred in 1983 and 1985.

> ➤ **Hlatky M, Boothroyd D, Vittinghoff E, Sharp P, and Whooley M (for the HERS Research Group).**

Quality-of-life and depressive symptoms in postmenopausal women after receiving hormone therapy (results from the Heart and Estrogen/Progestin Replacement Study (HERS) Trial. *Journal of the American Medical Association*, February 2002; 287:591–597. **Type:** Experimental (clinical trial)

Focus: An examination of the effect of HRT (combined therapy) on quality life and depression in postmenopausal women with diagnosed heart disease.

Conclusions: HRT has varying effects on the quality of life among postmenopausal women depending upon whether a woman has meno-pausal symptoms (e.g., hot flashes) or not. Women without a history of hot flashes had greater decline in physical measures, but women with hot flashes had improvements in quality of life measures.

Findings:

- Quality of life declined during follow-up for the entire cohort—both placebo group and HRT group.
- Both the placebo and HRT groups experienced physical and mental decline over a three year period, although depressive symptoms were not significantly changed.
- Women who received HRT (combined therapy) had a reduction in the frequency of hot flashes, vaginal dryness and sleep problems.
- Women who received HRT (combined therapy) had an increased frequency of vaginal discharge, uterine bleeding and breast symptoms.
- Women who had experienced hot flashes before starting HRT, had improved mental and physical health; women who did not have hot flashes before starting HRT had a greater decline in physical and mental health.
- HRT had significant negative effects on physical function, but it improved depressive symptoms.

Researchers' Comments: "These mixed results suggest that hormone therapy does not have a general benefit for postmenopausal women with heart disease; rather, it improves quality of life only for women with menopausal symptoms" (595).

Participants and Methods: Postmenopausal women (2763) with diagnosed heart disease formed the study group. The average age was 67 years. The study was a randomized, double blind, placebo-controlled clinical trial, the Heart and Estrogen/Progestin Replacement Study (HERS). Women were assigned to one of two treatment groups from 1993 to 1994: HRT group (conjugated equine estrogen, 0.625 mg/d + medroxyprogesterone acetate, 2.5 mg/d) or placebo. At baseline the women were assessed for general health, estrogen use, reproductive history and medical conditions. Quality of life questionnaires were completed by participants at baseline, four months, one year and annually thereafter. Analyses were restricted to the first three years of follow-up. Quality of life questionnaires assessed functional capacity, emotional health, vitality and depression. Physical function was assessed using the Duke Activity Status Index. Energy and fatigue was measures using a RAND scale. Mental health was measured using the RAND Mental Health Inventory. Depressive symptoms were assessed using a scale developed for the National Study of Medical Outcomes.

> ## Hunt K, Vessey M, McPherson K, and Coleman M.

Long-term surveillance of mortality and cancer incidence in women receiving hormone replacement therapy. *The British Journal of Obstetrics and Gynecology*, July 1987; 94:620–635. **Type:** Observational (cohort)

Focus: An investigation the effects of HRT on general mortality and cancer incidence.

Conclusions: Women who had used HRT had an increased incidence of endometrial cancer and breast cancer. There was no positive association for cervical cancer and the data for ovarian cancer was not significant.

Findings:

- An elevated incidence of breast cancer was found in women who had used HRT for a long duration **(*relative risk:* 1.59 for users/1.00 for nonusers)**.
- The effect of HRT on mortality was low.
- The incidence of endometrial cancer was significantly elevated among HRT users **(*relative risk:* 2.84 for users/1.00 for nonusers)**.
- The researchers found no elevated risk for ovarian cancer or cervical cancer in women who used HRT.

Researchers' Comments: "Data on breast cancer, while far from conclusive, do provide some cause for concern. We are worried about the high incidence of the disease in the face of low mortality" (633).

Participants and Methods: The subjects were 4544 women who were long-term users of HRT and who had attended menopause clinics in Great Britain before the end of 1982. The recruitment for the study started in 1978 and the study is still in progress. The women were questioned on risk factors, lifestyle, medical history, some social factors, menopause status and physical characteristics. Most of the women were 45–54 years of age at recruitment and during initial hormone use. The subjects were questioned in 1983 to obtain information of HRT use since participation in the study, to find the extent of morbidity and to gather missing baseline information. Because of problems in recruitment, some of it was done retrospectively.

> ## Kampen D and Sherwin B.

Estrogen use and verbal memory in healthy postmenopausal women. *Obstetrics and Gynecology*, June 1994; 83:979–983. **Type:** Observational (cohort)

Focus: An assessment of the difference in verbal memory in women receiving HRT and nonusers.

Conclusions: Estrogen affects memory in postmenopausal women.

Findings:

- Women who received HRT had higher scores on tests of immediate and delayed paragraph recall than nonusers.
- Estrogen users recalled more information from standardized short stores read to them, both immediately and following a 30-minute delay than did nonusers.
- No difference existed between the performance of users of HRT and nonusers on immediate or Delayed Pared Associates Test or on immediate or delayed recall of the Selective Reminding Test.
- No difference between users of HRT and nonusers appeared on a number of tests of cognitive functioning, including tests of spatial memory, language and attention span.
- Women who received combined therapy scored similarly to women who received estrogen alone.

Researchers' Comments: "In contrast to these positive findings for tests of secondary verbal memory, other cognitive functions did not seem to be affected by estrogen administration. This suggests that estrogen has a specific, and not a global, effect on cognition" (982).

Participants and Methods: In this Canadian study, 71 postmenopausal women (55 years or more) similar in socioeconomic characteristics, were recruited from the general population. Of the study group, 28 women were receiving HRT and 43 women were nonusers. However, nine of the 28 users of HRT had undergone a bilateral salpingo-oophorectomy and hysterectomy. Women were excluded if they had received drug therapy or psychotherapy for depression, had a history of heard injury, stroke, heart attack, alcoholism or had been postmenopausal for less than two years. Batteries of tests were administered to the women that measured verbal and spatial memory, functioning language, attention span and spatial skills. The women were assessed for general health, medical conditions, medications, reproductive history, blood estradiol levels and estrogen use (type and dosage). The women were assigned to one of two groups for analysis, those receiving HRT and the control group. HRT consisted of mostly conjugated equine estrogens and over half the women were taking combined therapy, estrogen plus progestin. The dosages ranged from 0.3 mg/d to 1.5 mg/d conjugated equine estrogen and 5mg/d to 10 mg/d medroxyprogesterone acetate. Other forms of HRT included esterified estrone, estradiol, estradiol valerate, estrone sulfate and estrone sulfate/piperazine plus megestrol acetate. Women had received oral, intravaginal, transdermal and intramuscular HRT.

➤ **Kritz-Silverstein D and Barrett-Connor E.**

Long-term postmenopausal hormone use, obesity, and fat distribution in older women. *Journal of the American Medical Association*, January 1996; 275:46–49. **Type:** Observational (cohort)

Focus: An investigation of long-term HRT and the development of obesity.

Conclusions: No association was found between long-term HRT use (15 years or more) and obesity. Users of HRT compared with nonusers, were similar in weight after 15 years; however, initially HRT users were leaner.

Findings:

• Women who used HRT had a lower baseline BMI (body mass index) than never users.

• No difference existed between users of HRT and nonusers on any follow-up measure of obesity, fat distribution or body composition.

• No significant association was found between the dosage of estrogen and obesity.

• Compared with nonusers, women who received HRT had the following characteristics: early age of menopause, exercised more regularly and drank alcohol three or more times a week.

• Women who had used HRT continuously or intermittently were more likely to have had a surgical menopause.

Researchers' Comments: "The Ranch Bernardo cohort is white, middle to upper-middle class, relatively well educated and at baseline was leaner than the US population. Therefore, these findings may not be generalizable to populations consisting of other racial, ethnic or socioeconomic groups" (48–49).

Participants and Methods: Between 1972 and 1974 a survey was initiated to determine the risk factors for heart disease in the southern California community of Rancho Bernardo. Between 1988 and 1991, 78 percent of the surviving women (65 years or older), participated in a follow-up clinic visit providing the data for this study. This study is based on 671 women (65–94 years old) who were either users, intermittent users or nonusers of HRT. All the women were postmenopausal at the beginning of this study. The average age of the 671 participants was 60.5 years. The women assessed for general health, medical conditions reproductive history, estrogen use, alcohol and cigarette consumption, physical exercise, body mass index and diet. Most of the women (98.6 percent) had received conjugated estrogen (Premarin) and only 18.8 percent had received combined therapy (estrogen + progestin). The most common dosage was 0.625 mg/d although some (15 percent) of the women 1.250 mg/d.

➤ Laya M, Larson E, Taplin S, and White E.

Effects of estrogen replacement on the specificity and sensitivity of screening mammography. *Journal of the National Cancer Institute,* May 1996; 88:643–649. **Type:** Observational (cohort)

Focus: An assessment of the effects of HRT on the accuracy (specificity and sensitivity) of mammograms.

Conclusions: Women who use HRT have an increase in density of breast tissue resulting in less sensitivity and accuracy in screening. This may result in decreased effectiveness of mammograms in these women.

Findings:

- The specificity of mammograms was lower in current users of HRT than in never or former users.
- *False-positive readings* in current users of HRT were higher than nonusers (**relative risk:** 1.33 for users/1.00 for nonusers).
- Women using HRT had a higher rate of *false-negative readings* that nonusers (**relative risk:** 1.09 for users/1.00 for nonusers).
- Thirty-one percent of the breast cancer in women who were current users of HRT was not detected by mammography and these false-negative cancers measured 15mm or more in diameter.
- Diagnostic accuracy of mammography was reduced in women receiving HRT.

Researchers' Comments: "An ERT-induced increase in mammographic density might result, therefore, in an increase in false-positive and/or false-negative readings among postmenopausal women" (644).

Participants and Methods: Participants in this study were postmenopausal women (50 years or more) enrolled in the Group Health Cooperative (GHC) of Puget Sound, Washington. This cooperative includes two hospital and twenty-one primary care facilities in western Washington State. The participants, compared with the general population, were better educated and more affluent. Through questionnaires, the women were assessed for general health, medical conditions, risk-factor history, mammogram screening history, reproductive history and estrogen use (type, duration, dosage). Most of the women were taking conjugated equine estrogen (Premarin). The women who were 50 years or older and selected women 40–49 years at high risk of breast cancer were asked to participate in a breast cancer screening program from 1988 to 1993. Women diagnosed with breast cancer within a year of the first screening were identified by the regional cancer registry.

➤ **LeBlanc E, Janowsky J, Chan B, and Nelson H.**

Hormone replacement therapy and cognition: systematic review and meta-analysis. *Journal of the American Medical Association*, March 2001; 285:1489–1499. **Type:** Statistical (meta-analysis)

Conclusions: Women who used HRT had a decreased risk of dementia; however, the studies had problems with methodology: possible biases and lack of control for potential confounding factors.

Findings:

- Based on data from observational studies, women who used HRT (estrogen) had a lower risk of dementia (*odds ratio:* 0.66 for users/ 1.00 for nonusers).
- HRT use was associated with improvement in some cognitive functions in women who had menopausal symptoms, but not in women without symptoms.
- Women who received HRT who had menopausal symptoms had improvements in verbal memory, reasoning and motor speed but no improvement in other cognitive functions.
- HRT did not affect visual recall, working memory, complex attention, mental tracking or verbal functioning.

Researchers' Comments: "HRT users might be less likely to develop Alzheimer disease not because of postmenopausal estrogen exposure but because they are healthier and have healthier lifestyles" (1497).

Participants and Methods: This meta-analysis examined studies of HRT and cognition from MEDLINE (1966–August 2000), HealthSTAR (1975–August 2000), PsychINFO (1984–August 2000), the Cochrane Library databases and referenced articles. Randomized controlled trials were analyzed for the effects of HRT on cognitive decline and observational studies were reviewed for the risk of dementia. Twenty-nine studies met inclusion criteria and were rated. The research did not assess the effects of progestin, different types of estrogen, doses or duration of therapy.

➤ **Marslew U, Overgaard K, Riis B, and Christiansen C.**

Two new combinations of estrogen and progestogen for prevention of postmenopausal bone loss: long-term effects on bone, calcium and lipid metabolism, climacteric symptoms and bleeding. *Obstetrics and Gynecology*, February 1992; 79:202–210. **Type:** Experimental (clinical trial)

Focus: An examination of the effects on bone, calcium, lipid metabolism, menopause symptoms and bleeding in women receiving HRT.

Conclusions: HRT (estrogen + progestin) prevents postmenopausal bone loss and results in a favorable lipid profile reducing the risk of cardiovascular disease.

Findings:

- HRT (combined therapy) with levonorgesterel produced more of a decrease in total cholesterol and low-density lipoprotein cholesterol than did combined therapy with *cyproterone acetate.*
- Both HRT treatment groups had a reduction in menopausal symptoms (e.g., hot flashes).
- Bone mineral density of the forearm during the two-year study remained unchanged in the HRT treatment groups, but decreased in the placebo group by 5 percent.
- Women who received HRT had a reduction in total cholesterol by 10 percent.
- No changes in HDL cholesterol were observed in the HRT groups or placebo group.
- The continuous regimen with cyproterone acetate resulted in 32 percent of the women reporting spotting; in the sequential regimen with *levonorgestrel* 84 percent of the women had regular bleeding.

Researchers' Comments: "Compliance with the treatments was about 5 percent lower than what we have experienced in previous studies. We ascribe this to the relatively high incidence of adverse effects, which eventually lead to 13 dropouts (17 percent); 12 women left the hormone groups whereas only one women left the placebo group"(207–208).

Participants and Methods: This Danish, two year small trial involved 62 postmenopausal women (45–54 years). The women were assessed for general health, medical conditions, medications, reproductive status and estrogen use. During the study, blood pressure, lipid profile, biochemical markers of bone turnover, weight changes, bone mineral density and menopausal symptoms were measured and monitored at three month intervals. Three treatment groups were formed: HRT (continuous estradiol valerate, 2 mg/d + cryproterone acetate, 1 mg/d), HRT (continuous estradiol valerate, 2 mg/d + sequential levonorgestrel, 75 μg 9 days) or placebo. Bone mineral density at various body sites was measured using dual-photon absorptiometry , dual-energy, X-ray absorptiometry and single-photon absorptiometry. The study was part double blind and part single-blind because of the impossibility of producing identical tablets.

➤ Medical Research Council's General Practice Research Framework

Randomized comparison of oestrogen versus oestrogen plus progestogen hormone replacement therapy in women with hysterectomy. *British*

Medical Journal, February 1996; 312:473–477. **Type:** Experimental (clinical trial)

Focus: A comparison of the symptomatic and metabolic effects of two hormone replacement therapies in women with hysterectomies.

Conclusions: Both treatments were approximately equal in terms of beneficial and adverse effects on lipid concentration and coagulation. Combined therapy (estrogen + progestogen) may be as cardioprotective as therapy with estrogen alone.

Findings:

• Estrogen alone and combined therapy led to a decrease in vasomotor symptoms (hot flashes and sweating).
• HDL levels were more elevated in the estrogen group than in the combined therapy group.
• Triglyceride levels were unchanged in the combined therapy group, and rose in the estrogen group.
• Fibrinogen concentration fell in both groups in but slightly more in the estrogen group.

Researchers' Comments: "When the study was initiated, it was thought that most women with a hysterectomy should take hormone replacement therapy. Hence no untreated (placebo) group was included" (473).

Participants and Methods: Three-hundred and twenty-one British women who had undergone hysterectomies (ages 35–59) participated in the study. This trial was conducted by seven group practices in the Medical Research Councils' general practice research framework. The recruitment was initiated in September 1991 and closed in March 1993. The results are based on follow-up until September 1994. Treatment consisted of two groups that were randomized and double blinded. These women were assessed for lifestyle, medical history, estrogen use, health habits, socioeconomic factors and menopause status. One group received estrogen and the other group received combined therapy (estrogen + progestogen).

➤ **Monster T, Janssen W, de Jong P, and de Jong-van den Berg L. (for the Prevention of Renal and Vascular End Stage Disease Study Group).**

Oral contraceptive use and hormone replacement therapy are associated with microalbuminuria. *Archives of Internal Medicine*, September 2001; 161:2000–2005. **Type:** Observational (case-control)

Focus: An investigation of the association between oral contraceptive use, hormone replacement therapy and microalbuminuria.

Conclusions: Long-term use of HRT or oral contraceptives increases a woman's risk of *microalbuminuria* and cardiovascular disease.

Findings:

- Postmenopausal use of hormone replacement was associated with an increased risk of microalbuminuria (**odds ratio:** 2.05 for users/1.00 for nonusers).
- Longer duration (5 years or more) of HRT was associated with an even higher risk of microalbuminuria (**odds ratio:** 2.56 for users/1.00 for nonusers).
- Premenopausal women who used oral contraceptives had an increased risk of microalbuminuria (**odds ratio:** 1.90 for uses/1.00 for nonusers).
- Higher estrogen content in oral contraceptives was associated with an increased risk of microalbuminuria.

Researchers' Comments: "Premenopausal oral contraceptive use and postmenopausal hormone replacement therapy are associated with a risk of cardiovascular disease.... Observational data show a beneficial effect of hormone replacement therapy on cardiovascular risk factors and mortality rates. Randomized clinical trials, however, do not support this beneficial role of hormone replacement therapy" (2000).

Participants and Methods: The data for this case-control study was obtained from the Prevention of Renal and Vascular End Stage Disease Cohort Study. The Participants (8592) were 28 to 75 years and resided in the Netherlands. Women from this study cohort (4301) formed the cases in this study. The participants were assessed for general health, menopausal status, tobacco use, body weight, blood chemistry, medical conditions, estrogen use, and oral contraceptive use. Pharmacy records of the participants were examined.

➤ **Mulnard R, Cotman C, Kawas C, van Dyck C, Sano M, Doody R, Koss E, Pfeiffer E, Shelia J, Gamst A, Grundman M, Thomas R, and Thal L.**

Estrogen replacement therapy for treatment of mild to moderate Alzheimer's disease. *Journal of the American Medical Association*, February 2000; 283:1007–1014. **Type:** Experimental (clinical trial)

Focus: An investigation of the effects of HRT on the global, cognitive or functional decline in women with mild to moderate Alzheimer's disease.

Conclusions: HRT (estrogen) for one year did not slow the progression of Alzheimer's disease in women who received therapy. This study does not support the use of estrogen as a treatment for Alzheimer's disease.

Findings:
- HRT did not improve the mental functioning in women who received therapy.
- 80 percent of the participants who received HRT worsened.
- 74 percent of the participants received the placebo worsened.
- Women who received HRT performed worse on the Clinical Dementia Rating Scale than the women who received the placebo.
- Women who received estrogen performed no better than the placebo on measures of cognitive, global or motor functioning.

Researchers' Comments: "Of public health concern is the tendency for experimental treatment to become standard of care before the rigorous scientific evidence is thoroughly gathered. Such is the concern with estrogen administration for women with AD" (1014).

Participants and Methods: The Alzheimer's Disease Cooperative Study was a twelve month, placebo-controlled, double blinded, randomized clinical trial. The participants, 120 women (greater than 60 years) with Alzheimer's disease and hysterectomies, were enrolled between October 1995 and January 1999. Thirty-two centers participated in the recruitment of the women. The women were assessed for general health, medical conditions, medications, reproductive history and estrogen use. Women were excluded from the study if they had a history of high cholesterol, heart disease, vascular disorders, estrogen use within the previous three months, and use of psychotropic medication. The participants were randomized to receive estrogen followed by a three month, placebo washout phase. The participants were allocated to one of three treatments: estrogen (0.625 mg/d), estrogen (1.25 mg/d) or placebo. Ninety-seven women completed the trial. Evaluation and follow-up occurred at two, six, twelve, and fifteen months. The researchers chose unopposed estrogens because previous investigations have suggested that progesterone may lessen some of estrogen's beneficial effects in the central nervous system. Measures of functioning included the Clinical Global Impression of Change (CGIC) 7-point scale and secondary measures (global, mood, cognitive).

▶ **Nachtigall L, Nachtigall R, and Beckman E.**

Estrogen replacement therapy II: A prospective study in the relationship to carcinoma and cardiovascular and metabolic problems. ***Obstetrics and Gynecology,*** July 1979; 54:74–79. **Type:** Experimental (clinical trial)

Focus: An examination the effects of HRT on postmenopausal women.

Conclusions: No increased incidence of breast cancer or endometrial cancer occurred with combined therapy (estrogen + progesterone). However, an increased incidence of gallstone formation was found in women who used HRT (combined therapy).

Findings:

- The estrogen treatment group had a significantly lower incidence of breast cancer than did the control group.
- Except for breast cancer, there was no statistically significant difference between groups for other disease related conditions.
- All HRT patients who started the study with an elevated *lipoprotein ratio* showed decreased levels within the first six months of treatment.
- Women who received HRT had a higher incidence of gallstone formation.
- The HRT group had a lower overall mortality rate.

Researchers' Comments: "These findings, however, should be interpreted with caution since the power of the test difference was generally low due to the small sample size" (76).

Participants and Methods: Four-hundred women were recruited at a hospital in New York City to participate in a trial. The trial was a ten-year prospective study, randomized and double blind. The women who participated were postmenopausal and had never undergone HRT. The women were assessed for general health, medical conditions, medications, reproductive history and estrogen use. Women who had heart disease and hypertension were excluded from the study. Eighty-four matched pairs were chosen according to age and other health related characteristics. Each member of a pair was randomly assigned to the treatment or control group. The final study group were matched for the major diagnosis. The most common diagnoses included diabetes mellitus, custodial care and arteriosclerosis. The remaining study groups were paired on the basis of chronic neurologic disorders. The treatment group received conjugated estrogen (2.5 mg/d) and medroxyprogesterone acetate (10 mg/d) for seven days a month. The control group received a placebo.

➤ **Paganini-Hill A.**

The benefits of estrogen replacement therapy on oral health. *Archives of Internal Medicine*, November 1995; 155:2325–2329. **Type:** Observational (cohort)

Conclusions: HRT may be beneficial in preventing tooth loss and the need for dentures in older women.

Findings:

• Women who had received HRT had significantly more teeth in each age group above 70 years.

• With increasing duration of HRT, there was decreasing tooth loss and denture wear.

• Dental health may benefit from HRT.

• Women using HRT had a lower risk for tooth loss than nonusers (*relative risk:* 0.81 for users/1.00 for nonusers).

Researchers' Comments: "The Leisure World population is a moderately affluent, well-educated and health conscious community" (2328).

Participants and Methods: A health survey questionnaire was mailed to all residents who owned homes in Leisure World Laguna Hills in June 1981. The response to the survey involved 13,979 residents forming the original cohort. The subjects were white, affluent, well educated and two-thirds women. The survey gathered information about medical history, lifestyle (smoking, alcohol consumption, exercise), health care use, reproductive history and HRT. A follow-up survey in November of 1992 assessed current health status. During this follow-up information was obtained regarding dental health. Female subjects (4,240) returned the questionnaire.

➤ **Parazzini F, LaVecchia C, Negri E, Franceschi S, Moroni S, Chatenoud L, and Bolis G.**

Case-control study of oestrogen replacement therapy and risk of cervical cancer, **British Medical Journal**, July 1997; 315:85–87. **Type:** Observational (case-control)

Focus: An examination of the relation between HRT and the risk of cervical cancer.

Conclusions: HRT does not increase the risk of cervical cancer.

Findings:

• Women who received HRT did not have an increased risk of cervical cancer (*odds ratio:* 0.50 for users/1.00 for nonusers).

• The risk of cervical cancer decreased with duration of use.

• The reduced risk of cervical cancer with HRT lasted for at least 10 years.

• Women who reported more sexual partners had a higher risk of cervical cancer.

• Women who had used oral contraceptives had a higher risk of cervical cancer than never users.

Researchers' Comments: "Women receiving oestrogen replacement therapy are screened more frequently than the background population" (87).

Participants and Methods: This hospital-based study involved 695 Italian women (40–75 years) in Milan, Italy. The women were diagnosed with invasive cervical cancer and admitted from 1981 to 1993 to the obstetrics and gynecology clinics of the University of Milan, the National Cancer Institute and the Ospedale Maggiore of Milan. The participants were assessed through questionnaires for information about HRT (type, dosage, duration), lifestyle (including alcohol, cigarette and coffee consumption) and medical history. The control group, 749 women (40 to 75 years) age-matched with cases, were hospitalized for conditions not related to cervical cancer, and were admitted to the same hospitals where the cases were selected. Women were excluded as controls if they were admitted for gynecological, hormonal or *neoplastic* conditions.

➤ **Polo-Kantola P, Portin R, Polo O, Helenius H, Irjala K, and Erkkola R.**

The effect of short-term estrogen replacement therapy on cognition: a randomized, double-blind, cross-over trial in postmenopausal women. *Obstetrics and Gynecology*, March 1998; 91:459–466. **Type:** Experimental (clinical trial)

Focus: An evaluation of the effect of short-term HRT (estrogen) on *cognitive* functioning.

Conclusions: Cognitive functioned decreased with age. Women who received HRT (estrogen) for a short duration did not perform cognitive tasks better than the women who received a placebo.

Findings:
- Performance on cognitive tasks decreased with increased age: older women were slower and made more errors than younger women.
- HRT (estrogen) did not improve a woman's performance on cognitive tasks.
- No correlation was found between cognitive performance and serum estrogen levels.
- Reaction times and error rates were not affected by serum estrogen levels.
- Performance tests scores generally were correlated to age: older women performed slower and made more errors than younger women.
- Cognitive performances were similar for past users and never users in the estrogen and placebo treatment groups.

Researchers' Comments: "Estrogen was not superior to the placebo in any task of our comprehensive test battery. In our present study with healthy and relatively young postmenopausal women, cognitive performance was well preserved. Furthermore, observed cognitive changes were mild, primarily age-related, and not reversible by ERT" (465).

Participants and Methods: This randomized, crossover trial (double blind/placebo controlled), conducted in Finland, involved 70 postmenopausal women (47 to 65 years) with previous hysterectomies. The women were recruited by a newspaper announcement. The women were assessed for demographic characteristics, general health, medical conditions, reproductive history, serum estrogen levels, estrogen use and medications. Women who had previously used HRT were accepted if they agreed to stop HRT for five months before the trial. The study design consisted of two three-month treatment periods dividing the women into two groups: group A received the placebo first and then estrogen; group B received estrogen first and then the placebo. Sixty-eight percent of the study group had used HRT before with average duration of use at 40 months. HRT consisted of transdermal estrogen, either gel (estrogen 2.5 g/d) or the patch (3.2 mg/d). The researchers administered cognitive tests measuring information processing, attention and working memory. Cognitive tests were given before estrogen treatment, at the end of each treatment and washout period.

➤ Raz R and Stamm W.

A controlled trial of intravaginal estriol in postmenopausal women with recurrent urinary tract infection. **The New England Journal of Medicine**, 1993; 329:753–756. **Type:** Experimental (clinical trial)

Focus: An examination of the effectiveness of estriol in the treatment of urinary tract infections.

Conclusions: Intravaginal estriol was found to be an effective preventive treatment for urinary tract infections in postmenopausal women.

Findings:

• Intravaginal estriol reduced the incidence of urinary tact infections compared with the placebo.

• Women who had received estriol remained free of urinary tract infections more than women who received the placebo.

• Women who received estriol had a drop in their vaginal pH (more acid) and therefore were less susceptible to infection.

• The placebo group did not have a drop in vaginal pH.

Glossary/Background Information: In premenopausal women, circulating estrogens contribute to the colonization of the vagina by lacto-bacilli, which produce lactic acid and maintain a low vaginal pH. This low pH inhibits the growth of yeast and other microorganisms. After meno-pause, the vaginal pH increases and in some women vaginal and urinary infections occur.

Researchers' Comments: "We studied topically applied estriol rather than the orally administered drug, since the former should be safer and should not produce systemic effects" (756).

Participants and Methods: The women enrolled in this trial (double blind/placebo-controlled) were 93 postmenopausal women. The women were patients treated at the Infectious Disease Clinic at Central Emek Hospital, Afula, Israel. All the patients were being treated for recur-ring urinary tract infections. The patents were assessed for general health, medical history, reproductive history, medications and estrogen use. Women were excluded from the study if they had any of the following con-ditions: thromboembolism disorders, liver disease, estrogen-dependent tumors, anatomical lesions in the urogenital area, an indwelling urinary catheter, a history of long-term use of antimicrobial agents for the pre-vention of urinary infections, or currently receiving oral estrogen therapy. Urine cultures were obtained at baseline, monthly (for eight months) and whenever urinary symptoms occurred. Vaginal cultures and pH measure-ments were obtained at baseline, at the first and the eighth month. The women were randomized to receive estriol topically applied as a intravagi-nal cream (50 women) or a placebo (43 women). Both of which were admin-istered intravaginally.

➤ **Rutter C, Mandelson M, Laya M, Seger D, and Taplin S.**

Changes in breast density associated with initiation, discontinuation, and continuing use of hormone replacement therapy. *Journal of the American Medical Association*, January 2001; 285:171–175. **Type:** Observational (cohort)

Focus: An examination of the effects of HRT on breast density in postmenopausal women.

Conclusions: Breast density is affected by HRT. HRT is associated with an increase in breast density. Discontinuation of therapy reduces breast density.

Findings:
• Women who start using HRT have an increase in breast density.
• Women who stop using HRT have a decrease in breast density.

- Women who continue to use HRT have a sustained increase in breast density.
- Women who use HRT have an increased risk of breast density (**relative risk:** 1.45 for users/1.00 for nonusers).
- Women who initiated HRT had increased breast density (**relative risk:** 2.57 for users/1.00 for nonusers).

Researchers' Comments: "Observed decreases in mammographic accuracy among women using HRT are a likely result of corresponding increases in density"(175).

Participants and Methods: The participants were 5212 postmenopausal women (40–96 years) enrolled in Group Health Cooperative (GHC) of Puget Sound, a health maintenance organization in western Washington State. The researchers obtained data from the breast cancer screening program initiated in 1985. The women were assessed for screening history, general health, menopausal status, HRT (type, dosage, duration) and risk factors. Eligible women were postmenopausal and had at least two screening examinations (mammograms) between 1996 and 1998. Women were excluded if they had a history of breast cancer, had a diagnosis of cancer before either screening, had a hysterectomy or underwent breast augmentation. Changes in breast density were coded into four groups: low density, decrease in density, increase in density and high density.

> ### Sanchez-Guerrero J, Liang M, Karlson E, Hunter D, and Colditz G.

Postmenopausal estrogen therapy and the risk for developing systemic lupus erythematosus. **Annals of Internal Medicine**, March 1995; 122: 430–433. **Type:** Observational (cohort)

Focus: The researches examined the relation between postmenopausal HRT and the development of systemic *lupus erythematosus.*

Conclusions: HRT is associated with an increased risk for developing systemic lupus erythematosus.

Findings:
- An increased risk of developing systemic lupus was found with longer duration HRT.
- Users of HRT had a greater risk for developing lupus than nonusers.
- Among users of HRT the risk for lupus was higher in current users than in past users.

Researchers' Comments: "Several potential limitations of this study must be considered. Because information on exposure to estrogen was based on self-reports, postmenopausal hormone use may have been misclassified.... Another potential source of bias is the possibility that increased opportunity for diagnosis of systemic lupus erythematosus might have occurred among women using hormones because they had to be under active medical care" (432).

Participants and Methods: The Nurses' Health Study cohort was initiated in June 1976. The participants, 69,435 female nurses, who had completed menopause and did not have Lupus or any other connective tissue disease. The women were recruited from eleven states and ranges in age for 30 to 55 years. These women were assessed for information on health, menopause status and HRT use. Follow-up information was gathered every two years until 1990. Questions about the diagnosis of Lupus were included in the 1982, 1984, 1986 and 1992 questionnaires. Medical records were obtained for all potential case of a systemic rheumatic disease. Definite cases of Lupus required at least four criteria. Since this strict criterion could potentially underestimate the true incidence of the disease, the researchers analyzed two other groups of patients: those meeting three or more criteria and those diagnosed by their physicians as having systemic lupus erythematosus even if they did not meet the four criteria.

➤ **Schaumberg D, Buring J, Sullivan D, and Dana M.**

Hormone replacement therapy and dry eye syndrome. *Journal of the American Medical Association*, November 2001; 286:2114–2119.
Type: Observational (cohort)
Focus: An investigation of the relationship between HRT and the development of *dry eye syndrome.*
Conclusions: Women who use HRT, particularly estrogen (alone) have an increased risk of developing dry eye syndrome
Findings:
• Women who received HRT (estrogen alone) had an increased risk of dry eye syndrome
• Women who received HRT (estrogen + progestin) had an increased risk of dry eye syndrome.
• For every three years of HRT there was a 15 percent increase in risk of dry eye syndrome.
Researchers' Comments: "Physicians caring for women who are taking or are considering HRT should be informed of the potential increased risk of dry eye syndrome with this therapy" (2119).
Participants and Methods: Data for this study was obtained from

the ongoing Women's Health Study, a randomized study of 25,665 post-menopausal women (aged 45 to 84 years) initiated in 1992 to evaluate the benefits and risk of aspirin and vitamin E in the prevention of cardiovascular disease and cancer. Participants complete annual questionnaires (baseline, 12 and 36 months) and report health-related information. At baseline the women were assessed for medical history, medical conditions, reproductive history, estrogen use, medications and supplement.

➤ **Seeley D, Cauley J, Grady D, Browner W, Nevitt M, Cummings S (for the Study of Osteoporotic Fractures Research Group).**

Is postmenopausal estrogen therapy associated with neuromuscular functions or falling in elderly women. *Archives of Internal Medicine,* February 1995; 155:293–299. **Type:** Observational (cohort)

Focus: An examination of the effect of postmenopausal estrogen use on muscle strength, neuromuscular functioning and risk of falling.

Conclusions: HRT did not have a beneficial effect on muscle strength or neuromuscular functioning, nor did it reduce the risk of falls.

Findings:
• No association was found between long term or short term estrogen use and muscular strength or functioning.
• Long term HRT users did not differ from short term users in strength or function.
• The dosage of estrogen was not associated with muscle strength or neuromuscular functioning.
• Current HRT users had isometric strength similar to that of never and past users.
• Current users of HRT had significantly lower hip and triceps strength than never or past users.

Researchers' Comments: "Although past users appear to have a lower risk of poor balance than never users, we cannot rule out the possibility that this is caused by selection bias, with healthier persons being past users of estrogens, or that it is a chance finding resulting form the number of statistical tests that were conducted" (298).

Participants and Methods: The study of Osteoporotic Fractures is a prospective study of risk fractures in older women. Recruitment occurred between September 1986 to October 1988. The Women were at least 65 years old from four US communities: Baltimore, Monongahela Valley (Pennsylvania), Portland and Minneapolis. Excluded from the study were black women because of their low incidence of hip fractures and women unable to walk without assistance or women with hip replacements. At baseline the women were questioned on the following factors: age, physical activity, diet, reproductive history, smoking, alcohol, caffeine intake, medical history, history of falls and fractures, medication and estrogen usage (dosage, duration and type). The women completed a physical exam including measurement of muscle strength, gait, balance and vision. The women also had their bone density measured. The researchers used six performance-based measures of function and self-reporting measures of disability and falls in the first year of follow-up. The six performance tests measured hip abductor, triceps extensor strength, hand-grip strength, standing balance, gait speed and timed chair stand.

➤ Selby P and Peacock M.

Dose dependent response of symptoms, pituitary, and bone to transdermal oestrogen in postmenopausal women. *British Medical Journal*, November 1986; 293:1337–1339. **Type:** Experimental (clinical trial)

Focus: An investigation of the effect of *transdermal* estrogen on bone tissue and menopausal symptoms in postmenopausal women.

Conclusions: Higher dosages of estrogen were more effective at relieving menopausal symptoms, but dosages above 150 pmol/l were not effective and may have an adverse effect by suppressing bone remodeling.

Findings:
- Transdermal estrogen was effective at relieving menopausal symptoms (hot flashes).
- Higher dosages of estrogen (up to 150 pmol/l) were more effective than lower dosages at relieving menopausal symptoms.
- HRT (transdermal estrogen) resulted in decreased excretion *urinary calcium.*
- HRT (transdermal estrogen) resulted in decreased excretion of *hydroxyproline.*

Researchers' Comments: "High doses of oestrogen have unwanted effects on bone as a result of inhibition of bone formation, which would be avoided by using the minimal dose of oestrogen to suppress resorption" (1337).

Participants and Methods: This small study (not blinded/no control group) conducted in England involved twenty-six postmenopausal women attending a clinic for menopausal symptoms. The women were assessed for general health, medical history and estrogen use. At baseline and at three weeks blood and urine analysis were done. These included follicle stimulating hormone levels, estrogen levels, urinary excretion of calcium, hydroxyproline and creatinine. Participants were randomly assigned to different sized patches of one of three treatment protocols: Transdermal estrogen (0.025 mg/d), transdermal estrogen (0.05 mg/d) or transdermal estrogen (0.1mg/d).

▶ **Shaywitz S, Shaywitz B, Pugh K, Fulbright R, Skudlarski P, Mencl W, Constable R, Naftolin F, Palter S, Marchione K, Katz L, Shankweiler D, Fletcher J, Lacadie C, Keltz M, and Gore J.**

Effects of estrogen on brain activation patterns in postmenopausal women during working memory tasks. *Journal of the American Medical Association*, April 1999; 281:1197–1202. **Type:** Experimental (clinical trial)

Focus: An investigation of the effects of estrogen on brain activation patterns in postmenopausal women performing memory tasks.

Conclusions: Estrogen alters brain activation patterns in postmenopausal women performing memory tasks. Estrogen affects brain organization for memory in postmenopausal women.

Findings:

• Estrogen therapy (1.25 mg/d) produced alterations in brain activation patterns in postmenopausal women as they performed working memory tasks.

• Estrogen did not affect performance of the women in verbal and non-verbal memory tasks.

Researchers' Comments: "A limitation of this study was the relatively brief time that women were receiving either estrogen or placebo and relatively short washout period between conditions" (1201)

Participants and Methods: This crossover trial from 1996 to 1998 (hospital setting) involved 46 right-handed, postmenopausal women who were 33 to 61 years of aged. The women were recruited for the study through posting in libraries, letters to women's group, physicians' offices and newspaper advertisements. The women were assessed for general health, medical conditions, medications, reproductive history and estrogen use. Participants were to meet the following criteria: having good general health, being right-handed, having normal structural magnetic resonance imaging findings, having an IQ of at least 85 and having the last menstrual period at least five months before entering the study. Women were excluded if they had *follicle-stimulating hormone* levels of 45 IU/L or less and estradiol levels that were at least 128pmol/L at baseline. The women did not receive any estrogen therapy for at least three months before the study. During the treatment protocol the women were randomized to receive estrogen or placebo. Participants were treated for two periods of 21 days each, one with conjugated equine estrogen (1.25 mg/d) and the other with an identical placebo with 14 days of washout between treatments. This study was blinded and placebo-controlled. Functional magnetic resonance imaging measured the effect of estrogen treatment in brain activation patterns during memory tasks. The stimuli for memory tasks were pronounceable nonsense words, and Tamil letters for the nonverbal memory tasks.

➤ Snabes M, Herd J, Schuyler N, Dunn K, Spence D, and Young R.

In normal postmenopausal women physiologic estrogen replacement therapy fails to improve exercise tolerance: A randomized, double-blind, placebo-controlled, crossover trial. *American Journal of Obstetrics and Gynecology*, July 1996; 175:110–113. **Type:** Experimental (clinical trial)

Focus: The objective of this study was to test whether estrogen replacement therapy could increase exercise tolerance in postmenopausal women.

Conclusions: Estrogen replacement therapy does not affect the blood flow to skeletal muscles or cellular oxygen use during exercise. Estrogen was not a vasodilator in the postmenopausal women in this study. Cardiovascular response was not improved with the use of HRT.

Findings:
- Systolic, diastolic, mean arterial and pulse pressures at rest and during treadmill exercises were not affected by estradiol treatment.
- Estradiol treatment did not change treadmill times or maximum oxygen uptake during exercise.
- The resting heart rate was lower in women receiving HRT.
- No positive effect from estrogen therapy was found on any ventilation parameter measured either during rest or during exercise.

Researchers' Comments: "A longer duration of treatment might be required to observe an effect of estradiol" (113).

Participants and Methods: This crossover-study involved thirty-one, healthy but sedentary postmenopausal women (55–65 years) who received 12 weeks of HRT (estradiol, 2 mg/d). The study was initiated by Baylor College of Medicine, Rice University at Houston Texas. The women were evaluated with Balke exercise treadmill tests. Four-hundred, seventy were screened, 36 were enrolled and 31 completed the study. The volunteers had no history of cardiac disease or systemic disease. Subjects had blood pressure equal to or less than 150/90 mm Hg. The women had blood analysis and complete physical exams including medical history. The participants were randomized to one of two treatment sequences. Fifteen women were given estradiol in period one and placebo in period two (sequence 1). Sixteen volunteers were given placebos in period one and estradiol in period two (sequence 2). Four exercise treadmill tests were performed. The baseline study was undertaken and then the procedure was repeated after 12 weeks of estradiol treatment. After a six-week washout, the participants had another exercise test as a second period baseline and after twelve weeks of treatment with placebo or estradiol, a final exercise test was given.

➤ Speroff L, Rowan S, Symons J, Genant H, and Wilborn W.

The comparative effect on bone density, endometrium, and lipids of continuous hormones as replacement therapy (Chart Study). *Journal of American Medical Association*, November 1996; 276:1397–1403.

Type: Experimental (clinical trial)

Focus: A comparison of the effect of continuous norethindrone acetate and ethinyl estradiol with unopposed ethinyl estradiol (estrogen alone) or placebo.

Conclusions: Combined therapy (*norethindrone acetate* + ethinyl estradiol) administered daily in low doses prevents proliferation of the endometrium, minimizes vaginal bleeding, assures a good lipid profile and provides an increase in bone mineral density. Triglyceride levels, however, were increased in women who used estrogen alone and in women who used combined therapy.

Findings:

- Bone mineral density increased more in women who used combined therapy than in women who used estrogen alone.
- Increased endometrial proliferation was found in women who received higher doses of unopposed estrogen (5 μg or more).
- The 10 μg treatment group which used ethinyl estradiol alone was terminated early because of an unacceptably high rate of endometrial hyperplasia.
- Continuous combined therapy increased HDL cholesterol and reduced LDL cholesterol.
- Both combined therapy and unopposed estrogen raised triglyceride levels in HRT users with higher levels appearing in women who used estrogen alone.
- Except for women receiving 10 micrograms of estrogen (ethinyl

estradiol), women who used unopposed estrogen did not have an increase in bone mineral density.

Researchers' Comments: "The placebo group had the smallest percentage of subjects reporting associated events ... for the other treatment groups, associated events appeared to be dose related" (1401).

Participants and Methods: This randomized clinical trial was conducted at 65 centers which enrolled 1,265 women subjects for outpatient treatment for two years. The women were assessed for general health, medical conditions, estrogen use, bone mineral density, blood chemistry and reproductive. The final treatment group enrolled at least 135 postmenopausal women, 40 years or older. All the participants were given calcium supplement and instructed to take 1000 mg daily in addition to their regular dietary intake of calcium. The women were randomized to placebo or one of eight treatment groups: (group 1) 0.2 mg of norethindrone acetate and 1 μg of ethinyl estradiol (group 2) 0.5 mg of norethindrone acetate and 2.5 μg of ethinyl estradiol (group 3) 1 mg of norethindrone acetate and 5 μg of ethinyl estradiol (group 4) 1 mg of norethindrone and 10 μg of ethinyl estradiol (group 5) 1 μg of ethinyl estradiol (group 6) 2.5 μg of ethinyl estradiol (group 7) 5 μg of ethinyl estradiol and (group eight) 10 μg of ethinyl estradiol. Reasons for being disqualified from the study included vaginal bleeding at baseline, baseline mammography indicative of cancer, chronic use of medications affecting calcium metabolism or vasomotor symptoms requiring medical intervention and noncompliance of HRT. There was a 22 percent dropout rate for the study.

▶ **Szklo M, Cerhan J, Diez-Roux A, Chambless L, Cooper L, Folsom A, Fried L, Knopman D, and Nieto J.**

Estrogen replacement therapy and cognitive functioning in the atherosclerosis risk in communities (ARIC) study. *American Journal of Epidemiology*, December 1996; 144:1048–1056. **Type:** Observational (cohort)

Focus: An assessment of the relation of HRT to cognitive functioning in postmenopausal women.

Conclusions: HRT was not associated with improved or higher level cognitive functioning in postmenopausal women. The overall patterns of cognitive scores did not indicate that HRT had a protective effect on mental abilities.

Findings:
• Among former HRT users, no clear associations were observed between duration of HRT and cognitive scores.

- Current users generally used HRT longer than former users and older women had used hormones longer than younger women.
- Current users of HRT were younger, better educated, more likely to be white, more often married and less frequently hypertensive or diabetic, had a lower body mass index, were less often smokers but more frequently consumers of alcohol.
- Among women ages 48 to 57 years, the mean WF test scores were slightly higher for HRT former and current users than for never users in both naturally and surgically menopausal women.

Researchers' Comments: "The current study, the largest to date, provides weak (if any) support for the hypothesis that ERT is independently related to cognitive functioning in postmenopausal women less than 67 years of age" (1054).

Participants and Methods: The study population involved postmenopausal women (48 to 67 years) who were participants in the Atherosclerosis Risk in Communities (ARIC) Study. The ARIC study is a prospective investigation of atherosclerosis in following communities: Jackson, Mississippi, selected Minneapolis suburbs, Minnesota, Forsyth County, North Carolina and Washington County, Maryland. A baseline examination of the cohort occurred in 1987 to 1989, and a follow-up examination from 1990 to 1992. From this cohort, 6,110 women participated in cognitive functioning tests: the Delayed Word Recall (DWR) Test, the Digit Symbol Subtest of the Wechsler Adult Intelligence Scale-Revisited (DSS/WAIS-R) and the Word Fluency (WF) Test of the Multilingual Aphasia Examination.

➤ **Weinstein L, Bewtra C, and Gallagher J.**

Evaluation of a continuous combined low-dose regimen of estrogen-progestin for treatment of the menopausal patient. *American Journal of Obstetrics and Gynecology,* June 1990; 162:1534–1542. **Type:** Experimental (clinical trial)

Focus: An evaluation of the effectiveness of low-dose combined therapy (estrogen + progestin) in the treatment of menopausal conditions.

Conclusions: Continuous low-dose combined therapy (estrogen + progestin) is effective in dealing with menopausal symptoms (e.g., hot flashes, vasomotor symptoms) improve cardiovascular health by raising HDL cholesterol and lowering LDL cholesterol and protects the endometrium form neoplasia.

Findings:
- Women receiving low-dose combined therapy (0.625 mg/d conjugated

estrogen + 2.5 mg/d or 5 m/dg of medroxyprogesterone acetate) had less withdrawal bleeding after 26 weeks of HRT.
- No clinical difference was found between the 2.5 mg and 5 mg doses of progestin (medroxyprogesterone acetate).
- Total cholesterol decreased in the women receiving continuous combined therapy, but this was not statistically significant.
- HDL cholesterol increased in women receiving low-dose continuous combined therapy.
- Triglyceride levels and very-low density lipoprotein cholesterol increased in all women receiving continuous combined therapy.

Researchers' Comments: "It is our opinion that the use of sequential regimen of estrogen-progestin does not increase the risk of breast cancer. The impact of continuous low-dose regimen of estrogen-progestin on the incidence of breast cancer risk is unknown, but we believe that it is unlikely to be increased" (1538).

Participants and Methods: This small, year long clinical trial involved 92 postmenopausal women. The women were evaluated at baseline for medical and reproductive history They were also evaluated with pelvic exams, endometrial biopsies, Papanicolaou smears, mammograms, urinanalysis and blood analysis. Vasomotor symptoms, vaginal bleeding and other menopausal side effects were tabulated by reference to daily diaries kept by the study's participants. At three, six, nine and twelve months the women were also given physical examinations, an evaluation of their diaries, and an analysis of lipoproteins in their blood. At six months the women were also assessed for blood count, liver functioning, and glucose levels. The participants were randomly assigned to two treatment groups: forty-six women received conjugated equine estrogen (0.625 mg/d) + medroxyprogesterone acetate (2.5 mg/d); forty-six women received conjugated estrogen (0.625 mg/d) + medroxyprogesterone acetate (5 mg/d). Both regimens were administered as continuous combined HRT.

➤ Weiss N, Daling J, and Chow W.

Incidence of cancer of the large bowel in women in relation to reproductive and hormonal factors. *Journal of the National Cancer Institute*, July 1981; 67:57–60. **Type:** Observational (case-control)

Focus: An investigation the effects of reproductive and hormonal factors on the development of large bowel cancer in women.

Conclusions: Events during a woman's reproductive life can affect her risk of developing *colon cancer.*

Findings:

- HRT (estrogen) was not associated with an increased risk of colon or rectal cancer.
- Women who had colon cancer had given birth to fewer children than the controls.
- Age at first birth, had no relationship to the occurrence of colon or rectal cancer.
- Oral contraceptive use was associated with an increased risk of rectal cancer but not colon cancer; however, the risk was not statistically significant.
- The incidence of colon cancer was reduced by 50 percent in women who had three or more children.

Researchers' Comments: "A mechanism by which pregnancy per se might act to protect against the development of colon cancer is through a decrease in bile acid secretion into the intestinal tract" (60).

Participants and Methods: Participants for this study were Caucasian women recruited in 1977 using the Cancer Surveillance System, a population cancer reporting system in Washington state. The cases were women (35 to 74 years) who had a diagnosis of colon cancer or rectal cancer during a 15-month period in 1976 to 1977. The controls, derived from the same population, were age-matched with cases. The cases were similar to the control group in income and marital status. The cases were, however, taller and leaner than the control group. All the participants were assessed for general health, medical conditions, reproductive history, estrogen use and medications.

➤ **Yaffe K, Sawaya G, Lieberburg I, and Grady D.**

Estrogen therapy in postmenopausal women: Effects on cognitive function and dementia. *Journal of the American Medical Association*, March 1998; 279:688–695. **Type:** Statistical (meta-analysis)

Focus: An examination of the effects of postmenopausal HRT on cognitive function and *dementia.*

Conclusions: HRT (estrogen) improves cognitive skills and reduces a woman's risk of dementia; however, current research is weak in methodology and is conflicting in results. Because of the inconclusive data and the risks associated with HRT (e.g., endometrial abnormalities, gallbladder disease, thromboembolic events and breast cancer), the researchers advise against HRT for the treatment of Alzheimer's disease.

Findings:

- Evidence exists that estrogen may improve cognitive functioning in postmenopausal women with symptoms; however, no conclusive evidence suggests that asymptomatic women would benefit from treatment.

- A largest observational study with sound methodology did not find any benefit from estrogen for treatment of dementia.
- The results of eight small trials on estrogen therapy in women without dementia are inconclusive.
- Weak evidence for the benefit of estrogen is found in the observational studies; these studies are susceptible to confounding and compliance bias.
- Only 58 women have been studied in clinical trials of the effect of HRT (estrogen) on Alzheimer's disease and these trials are mostly uncontrolled, unblinded and nonrandomized.
- Meta-analysis of ten observational studies showed a 29 percent decreased risk of developing dementia among estrogen users; however, the studies are small, and have study design problems.

Researchers' Comments: "Given the known risk of estrogen therapy, we do not recommend estrogen for the prevention or treatment of *Alzheimer disease* or other dementias until adequate trials have been completed" (688).

Participants and Methods: The researchers conducted a computerized MEDLINE search from January 1966 through June 1997, manually searched bibliographies of selected articles and consulted experts to obtain data for this analysis. The researchers included those studies that evaluated the biological mechanisms of estrogen's effect on the central nervous system and studies dealing with the effect of estrogen on cognitive functioning or dementia. Excluding case reports and studies of premenopausal women, 27 studies were reviewed. Of these, 13 dealt with the effect of estrogen on cognitive functioning and 10 examined the effect of estrogen on the risk of developing Alzheimer's disease or other dementia.

➤ **Zandi P, Carlson M, Plassman B, Welsh-Bohmer K, Mayer L, Steffens D, and Breitner J (for the Cache County Memory Study Investigators.)**

Hormone replacement therapy and incidence of Alzheimer's disease in older women (The Cache County Study). *Journal of the American Medical Association*, November 2002; 288:2123–2129. **Type:** Observational (cohort)

Focus: An investigation of the relationship between HRT and the risk of developing Alzheimer's disease in a group elderly women.

Conclusions: Women who had used HRT in the past had a reduced risk of developing Alzheimer's disease. Current use of HRT was associated with a reduced risk of the disease if a woman had used hormones for more than ten years.

Findings:

- The development of Alzheimer's disease (AD) was more common in women than men.
- Alzheimer's disease was less common in women who had used HRT.
- For women more than eighty years of age, the risk of developing AD was twice that of men.
- Women who had received HRT had a reduced risk of AD compared with nonusers.
- Women who had used HRT for more than ten years had a risk for AD similar to men (**hazard ratio:** 0.77 of users).
- Past users of HRT had a reduced risk of AD, but current users had a reduced risk of AD if they used HRT for more than 10 years (**hazard ratio:** 0.32 for past use 3–10 years/2.12 for current use 3–10 years/ 0.55 for current use of more than ten years.

Researchers' Comments: "Our observations suggest that the benefits of HRT, if any, may take years to appear, and a considerable latency period may intervene between treatment and perceptible effect" (2129).

Participants and Methods: The Cache Country Study is a prospective cohort study initiated in 1995 in Utah involving 5677 older residents (2928 women) of the Cache country. The participants, sixty-five years and older, were assessed for general health, medical conditions, apolipoprotein genotype, hormone use, medications, mental and neurological functioning. Tests of mental evaluation included the Modified Mini-Mental State examination, Dementia Questionnaire, neuropsychological tests. Of the participants, 1066 women (56.4 percent) reported use of HRT with an average exposure of 11.6 years. These users were younger and more educated than nonusers. From all the study participants the researchers initially identified 152 individuals with dementia (98 women, 54 men). During the three-year follow-up from 1998 to 2000, thirty-three new cases (25 women, 8 men) were diagnosed.

Glossary

adenocarcinoma: a malignant growth (cancer) derived from glandular tissue; tumor cells form recognizable glandular structures

alendronate (Fosamax): a bisphosphonate used to inhibit bone loss and increase bone density in postmenopausal women; not recommended for women with stomach or kidney problems; irritates the esophagus if not taken correctly

alkaline phosphatase: an enzyme; high levels are a marker of bone turnover

Alzheimer's disease: a degenerative disorder of the brain, involving progressive atrophy of intellectual and emotional functions; loss of the ability to process and retain information; thought to be a result of malfunctioning neuron fibers in the brain and the formation of abnormal protein plaques in aging adults

androgen: one of the three types of gonadal steroids found in both males and females

androstenedione: an androgen

angina: pain or tightness in the chest associated with artery blockage and heart disease

angiography: a technology (radiographic) used to visualize blood vessels for diagnosing coronary artery disease

apolipoproteins (lipoprotein a): a plasma lipoprotein similar to low-density lipoproteins (LDL cholesterol); a risk factor for coronary heart disease

arteriosclerosis: a group of diseases characterized by thickening and loss of elasticity of the artery walls

association: a statistical relationship of dependence between two or more variables; strength of the observed relationship is a criterion for evaluating whether a factor causes a disease

atherosclerosis: a common form of arteriosclerosis in which deposits of yellowish plaques containing cholesterol appear in arteries

autonomic system: self controlling; refers to the autonomic nervous system including the heart, smooth muscles and glands

baseline: the beginning of the study

benign breast disease: lumpy or fibrocystic breast thought to result from hormonal fluctuations; common enough in women so that the condition is not really a disease

bilateral oophorectomy (bilateral salpingo-oophorectomy): surgical removal of the ovaries and fallopian tubes; often performed with a hysterectomy

biliary tract surgery: pertaining to the gallbladder or bile ducts

bisphosphonate: a drug that prevents bone loss by blocking the activity of cells (osteoclasts) that breakdown bone tissue

blood pressure (diastolic): a measure of blood pressure (lower number); the stage of the heart cycle in which the heart muscle is relaxed, allowing the chamber to fill with blood

blood pressure (systolic): a measure of blood pressure (higher number); the stage of the heart beat when the heart contracts and the chambers pump blood during the heart cycle

breast cancer: abnormal growth and proliferation of cells in breast tissues; usually starts in the lining of the milk ducts as a precancerous condition (DCIS, ductal carcinoma in situ); if these cells leave the ducts and invade other tissue, metastasis occurs with the breast cancer cells invading the blood vessels and spread to other organs; risk and incidence for breast cancer increases with age (approximately 1 in 223 for a 40-year-old woman and 1 in 8 for 85-year-old woman); only 5 to 10 percent of breast cancer cases result from genetics, BRCA1 or BRCA2 genes may be involved; hypotheses for risks for developing breast cancer include lifetime exposure to estrogen and progesterone (endogenous and exogenous sources), early menarche and late menopause, environmental assault and lifestyle (high fat diet and obesity, lack of exercise, exposure to chemicals, alcohol, and tobacco), radiation therapy, nullparity; average age for breast cancer is 69 and one-third of women diagnosed with breast cancer will die of the disease

breast density: thick, dense breasts; reduce the accuracy of mammograms because the tissue can hide the visibility of cancer and other growths; HRT increases breast density

C-reactive protein: a blood protein that is a marker for inflammation and is associated with an increased risk cardiovascular disease

carcinoma: a malignant growth made up of epithelial cells often invading the surrounding tissues resulting in metastases

cardiovascular: pertaining to the heart and blood vessels

cardiovascular disease: heart disease, myocardial infarction, stroke, hypertension, hyperlipidemia, diabetes or peripheral vascular disease and stroke; disease of the blood vessels; narrowing of the blood vessels because of spasm or plaque formation and insufficient delivery of blood to the organs such as the heart and brain; risks include smoking, obesity, sendentary lifestyle, high cholesterol and triglycerides, diet high in animal fats, high blood pressure, arterial inflammation, viral and bacterial infections, diabetes; highest mortality of diseases that afflict men and women

carotid artery: principal artery in the neck; carries blood from the heart to the capillaries; composed of three layers (externa, media and intima); when impaired by the disease atherosclerosis, the risk of blood clot formation increases because plaques that appear on the inner walls of arteries reduces the blood flow through the arteries; ultrasonic measurements of this artery in the neck are used to assess the composition of the various layers and a person's risk of heart disease; aging is associated with a reduction of elastic fibers and smooth fibers in the media layer of the carotid artery

case-control studies: cases (with the disease) and controls (without the disease) are examined for their prior history of exposure; past exposure is compared between those who now have the disease and those who do not

cerebral: pertaining to the cerebrum, the main portion of the brain, occupying the upper part of the skull

cerebrovascular: pertaining to the blood vessels of the brain

chlorotrianisene: an estrogenic compound used for HRT

cholesterol: a kind of lipid; functions to build cell membranes, brain and nerve tissues and is the starting molecule for steroid hormones needed for metabolic regulation

cholesterol (HDL): a fat measured as part of total cholesterol; called good cholesterol because it functiins as a carrier, removing excess cholesterol from the artery walls

cholesterol (LDL): a fat measured as part of total cholesterol; called bad cholesterol because it is deposited on the artery walls; higher LDL levels arc associated with a higher risk of heart disease

cognitive: mental processes

cohort: a group made up of individuals of the same generation or age

cohort studies: investigates a group of people prospectively for the development of disease who have been exposed and not exposed to a factor (e.g., hormones, chemicals)

colon cancer: abnormal proliferation of tissue in the lower intestinal tract; the third most diagnosed cancer in women; screening recommended at age fifty; if caught early, it is treatable (90 percent 5-year survival) if the tumor is caught when it is local, but survival decreases to about 6 percent if metastasis has occurred

colorectal cancers: cancers of the rectum and colon

combined therapy: includes progestogen with estrogen and as a form of HRT to reduce the risk of endometrial cancer

conclusions: generalizations and inferences based on the findings of a study

confidence interval: a statistical range of values with a lower and upper limit and a degree of confidence (usually 95 percent); the two limits contain the parameter of the sample

confounding factors (variables): variables that can affect the outcome of a study and need to be controlled for in the research design or by statistics

conjugated equine estrogen: a mixture of sodium salts of the sulfate esters of estrogenic substances, usually estrone and equilin (e.g., Premarin); derived from pregnant mares' urine and is frequently used in HRT either alone or in combined therapy with progestin

continuous combined therapy: hormone replacement therapy in which estrogen and progestin are used together simultaneously throughout the monthly cycle; usually no menstrual cycle occurs with this regimen

continuous estrogen therapy with cyclical progestin therapy: estrogen is taken every day and progestin is taken from the 1st to 12th of each month

coronary angiography: catheter is inserted through the vessels leading to the heart and dye is injected in order to visualize and x-ray the arteries using a special camera

coronary artery occlusion: obstruction of the coronary artery, usually a result of plaque formation; sometimes complicated by thrombosis (blood clots)

coronary calcification: the buildup and formation of calcium plaques in the arteries resulting in disease of the arteries (atherosclerosis) *coronary event:* coronary death and nonfatal heart attack

coronary heart disease: disease of the arteries that supply blood to the heart muscle; symptoms include chest pain associated with exercise, shortness of breath, pain radiating down the left arm or to the jaw; more severe pain associated with nausea, vomiting, sweating and feeling faint; symptoms of a heart attack also include chest pain associated with exercise

cortical: hard outer part of the bones

cross-sectional study: uses a survey to gather data on a study group or groups about exposure to some risk factor and health outcomes; often involves participants who are questioned about a particular symptom or symptoms at a given moment in time; are broad in scope, uncomplicated in their design; are economical, provide large samples and yield rapid results; give information about a particular group, but cannot explain why a symptom or factor exists and cannot determine cause and effect; require human and time resources and lack depth of other study designs

cyclical hormone therapy: estrogen is taken days 1 through 25 and progestin is added for the last 10 to 14 days, usually followed by 5 or 6 days of no therapy; menstrual periods often occur with this regimen

cyproterone acetate: a synthetic progestin used in combination with estrogen for HRT

dementia: mental deterioration

densitometry: a tool used to measure bone density; variations in density are determined by comparison with another material or certain standards

deep vein thrombosis: blood clot in a vein often in a leg

diastolic blood pressure: a measure of blood pressure (lower number); the stage of the heart cycle in which the heart muscle is relaxed, allowing the chamber to fill with blood; residual pressure between heart beats

diethylstilbestrol (DES): a chemical complex that acts like estrogen; used for regulation of the menstrual cycle, in contraceptives, and to prevent premature labor; implicated in cervical cancer in daughters of pregnant mothers given DES

dilation and curettage: surgical scrapping of the lining of the uterus

distal forearm: the forearm furthest away from the body

distal radius: forearm

dry eye syndrome: a condition of the eye resulting in damage to the ocular surface and symptoms of dryness and irritation; associated with an increased risk of corneal infection; can cause permanent visual impairment in severe cases

dual energy x-ray absorptiometry (DEXA): measures bone density of the spine, hip and total body; can detect a loss of 1 percent of bone mass per year; a decrease of one standard deviation (approximately 10 percent bone loss) doubles the fracture risk and 2.5 standard deviations below the mean indicates significant osteoporosis; measures only lumbar spine not the upper back and it cannot detect fractures such as crush fractures in the vertebrae

dual-photon absorptiometry: measures total cortical and trabecular bone mineral content of the hip and spine

ductal carcinoma in situ (DCIS): an early, noninvassive breast cancer that has not metastasized (invaded) surrounding or peripheral tissue or organs; surgery depends on whether the cancer developed in a duct or a lobule

dyspnea: difficult or labored breathing

embolism: sudden blocking of an artery by a clot or foreign material brought to the site by the bloodstream

emulsification: the process in which bile salts coat tiny fat droplets and keep them from coalescing

endogenous: developing or originating within the body; growing from within

endogenous estrogens: estrogens that are naturally produced in the body

endometrial biopsy: removal of tissue from the endometrium for analysis

endometrial cancer: abnormal growth and uncontrolled proliferation of the lining of the uterus; associated with estrogen alone therapy or endogenous sources of estrogen unopposed by progesterone; risks include obesity, infertiltiy and irregular periods; symptoms include abnormal bleeding or postmenopausal bleeding; high survival rate if diagnosed early

endometrioid ovarian cancer: a type of epithelial ovarian cancer

endometrial hyperplasia: abnormal growth or cellular changes in a woman's endometrium

endometrioid carcinomas: cancer of the endometrium

endometrium: the inner lining of the uterus

end points: the parameter measured to answer the most important question of the clinical trial; types include measurements of quality of life, length of survival, disease rates, complication rates, intermediate measures (e.g., symptoms)

epithelial ovarian cancer: a type of ovarian cancer involving uncontrolled abnormal growth of the surface tissue of the ovary; typed as serous, mucinous, endometroid, Brenner, or clear cell tumors; classified as benign, borderline or malignant; malignant forms are called ovarian adenocarcinomas

epithelial ovarian tumors: cancerous growths on the surface of the ovary that do not usually become malignant; often called borderline tumors

esterified estrogen: a mixture of sodium salts of esters of estrogenic substances, principally estrone; used in HRT

estradiol: naturally occurring estrogen in humans; used in HRT often obtained from animal sources (hog ovaries and urine of pregnant mares); also prepared synthetically

17β-estradiol: form of estrogen used in many estrogen patches

estradiol valerate: a synthetic estrogen used mostly in Europe in HRT

estriol: a naturally occurring, weak human estrogen; a metabolic product of estradiol and estrone found in the urine; endometrial hyperplasia and postmenopausal vaginal bleeding are not associated with this estrogen; mainly converted in the liver from estrone and also estradiol; used in HRT primarily in Europe; high doses required to alleviate menopausal symptoms so some physicians have used estriol in combination with other estrogens (80 percent estriol, 10 percent estrone and 10 percent estradiol)

estrogen: primary female steroid sex hormones, which are produced in the ovary by the developing follicle; maintains the female reproductive system and develop secondary female sex characteristics; causes deposits of fat in breasts and hips, increases water retention, affects calcium metabolism, stimulates breast development and promotes sexual development; used primarily in oral contraceptives and in HRT

estrogenic: an adjective referring to the activity and effects of estrogen

estrogen-receptor negative tumors: tumor cells that are not stimulated by estrogen to grow

estrogen receptor–positive breast cancer: cell receptors in breast cancer tissue that respond positively to estrogen and result in abnormal proliferation of breast tissue cells

estrogen receptor status: breast cancer tissue that proliferates in response to estrogen

estrone (E1): occurs naturally in pregnancy urine, in the human placenta and in palm kernel oil; also prepared synthetically; estrone is converted in the body from androstenedione or estradiol; orally administered estrogens include estrone, combinations of estrone and estradiol or estradiol alone

estrone sulfate: a type of synthetic estrogen used in HRT

ethinyl estradiol: a synthetic estrogen used in HRT and oral contraceptives; naturally occurring estradiol is the most potent form of estrogen in the body; when used for contraception it is formulated with progestin; used in HRT in lower doses with norethidrone acetate a (progestin)

etiologies: causes

etidronate: a bisphosphonate used to treat osteoporosis

experimental studies: clinical trials; involves randomization and double blind study design; examines effects of an independent variable on a dependent variable (e.g., effects of HRT on cardiovascular disease)

exogenous: originating outside the body

factor: a voluntary or involuntary environmental exposure such as a medication, a hormone, a chemical, a food, alcohol and cigarettes

false-negative readings: an incorrect reading of abnormal breast tissue as normal

false-positive readings: an incorrect reading of normal breast tissue as abnormal

femoral neck: the point where the thigh bone connects with the pelvis; connection between upper leg and hip

femur: thigh bone; the leg bone extended from the pelvis to the knee

fibrin: a protein formed during normal clotting of the blood

fibrinogen: a plasma protein converted to fibrin; involved in blot clot formation

fibrinolysis: dissolving fibrin in the blood

fibrinolytic: the destruction of the protein fibrin (a component of blood clots) by enzymes

findings: date gathered, analyzed and presented in a study

follicle stimulating hormone (FSH): produced by the pituitary gland; stimulates the ovaries to produce estrogen; promote maturation of the follicle; levels of FSH are elevated after menopause and sometimes during perimenopause

gallbladder disease: bile which is produced in the liver and plays a role in the emulsification of fat is stored in the gallbladder; disease of the gallbladder involves inflammation and abdominal pain; the formation of stones within the gallbladder (cholelithiasis) occurs and can result in obstruction of the duct; tumors can also be a problem and can be asymptomatic until they have extended into the liver or cause obstruction

gestagen: European term for progestin

globulin: a class of proteins; higher serum concentrations bind and inactivate estradiol increasing the risk of hip and vertebral fractures.

glucose: a sugar measured as part of blood chemistry

gonadotropins (FSH, LH): hormones that affect the ovaries in females;

decreased levels during menopause stimulate the secretion of follicle stimulating hormone or luteinizing hormone by the pituitary gland to compensate for the deficiency

gynaecological (British spelling): pertaining to gynecology, the branch of medicine that treats conditions and diseases affecting a woman's reproductive system

gynecological (American spelling): pertaining to gynecology, the branch of medicine that treats conditions and diseases affecting a woman's reproductive system

hazard ratio: relative risk

HDL cholesterol: a fat measured as part of total cholesterol; often called good cholesterol because it functions as a carrier, removing excess cholesterol from the walls of the arteries

heart rate variability (HRV): a statistical measure of the cyclic beat-to-beat variation heart rate; reduced HRV is an independent marker for an increased risk of mortality after a heart attack

hydroxproline: an amino acid obtained from urine used as a biochemical indicator of bone turnover and bone loss

hyperparathyroidism: refers to the condition of an abnormal increase in the activity of the parathyroid glands (near the thyroid glands which are located on the surface of the trachea); parathyroid hormones are involved in the metabolism of calcium and phosphorus from bone; they also increase reabsorption of calcium and excretion of phosphorus by the kidney; excess parathyroid hormones results in adverse functioning of bone cells, kidney tubules and mucus membranes of the stomach and intestines; the development of kidney stones and calcium deposits in the kidney tubules and decalcification of the bones (osteoporosis)can occur

hyperplasia: the abnormal multiplication or increase in the number of normal cells in a tissue

hypercholesterolemia: high blood levels of cholesterol usually greater than 250 mg/dl

hypertension: elevated blood pressure

hypertensive: high blood pressure usually measured as systolic pressure greater than 140mm and diastolic pressure greater than 90mm

hypertriglyceridemia: high levels of triglycerides in the blood

hypoestrogenic: premature ovarian failure or pituitary tumor

hypothesis: theory; an assumption made in order to test its consequences

hysterectomy: surgical removal of the uterus

idiopathic: self originating; unknown causation

incidence: the measurement of the rate at which people without a disease develop the disease during a given period; number of new cases of a disease during a given time divided by the population at risk of developing the disease

incidence rate: the measure of the number of new cases of a disease over a period of time divided by the population at risk of developing the disease

in situ: confined to the site of origin without invasion to other tissues

insulin: regulates blood sugar and plays a role in fat metabolism; increases cholesterol synthesis

interluekin-6: elevated levels in the blood indicate inflammation and an increased risk for heart attack and other cardiovascular conditions *intimal-medial carotid:* refers to the inner layers of the carotid artery

invasive ductal carcinoma: cancer of the breast ducts that can spread (metastasize) to other organs

invasive lobular carcioma: cancer of the breast lobule that can spread (metastasize) to other organs

in vitro: observable in a test tube

in vivo: within a living body

ischemic heart disease: deficiency of blood in the heart due to constriction or obstruction of a blood vessel; coronary heart disease

isometric: exercises in which one muscle is employed against another or against an immovable object

latency period: time span for the development of a disease

LDL cholesterol: a fat measured as part of total cholesterol; called bad cholesterol because it is deposited on the artery walls; higher LDL levels are associated with a higher risk of heart disease

LDL1 cholesterol: large, light particles thought to accumulate easily in the bloodstream; their oxidation may contribute to atheroscerolsis (clogging of the arteries)

LDL2 cholesterol: small, heavy cholesterol particles

LDL lipoproteins: small and large LDL particles composed of protein and fat; lipoproteins; found in the bloodstream and function as cholesterol carriers; comprised of a number of subclasses

levenorgestrel: a type of progestin used in combination with estrogen in HRT

lipids: fats; group of organic substances that are insoluble in water but soluble in alcohol, ether, chloroform and other fat solvents

lipoproteins: made of fats and proteins; found in the bloodstream and function as cholesterol carriers

lipoprotein (a): a plasma lipoprotein similar to low-density lipoproteins (LDL cholesterol); a risk factor for coronary heart disease

lipoprotein ratio: the ratio of HDL cholesterol to total cholesterol

lobular breast cancer: abnormal proliferation of the cell in the breast lobes

lobular carcinoma in situ (LCIS): a localized form of breast cancer often associated with micro calcifications; small flecks of calcium found in areas of rapid cell divisions

long-cycle hormone replacement therapy: a therapy of unopposed estrogen for two to six months between progestin treatments

lumin: the channel within the blood vessel or artery

lupus erythematosus: a disease in which large scale production of autoantibodies result in an individual's immune system attacking itself; all organs and DNA can be affected

mastalgia: pain in the mammary glands (breasts)

medroxyprogesterone acetate: a progestin (synthetic progesterone) used in combination with estrogen in HRT to causes the shedding of the uterine lining helping to prevent endometrial cancer; side effects include symptoms of PMS such as headaches, depression, irritability, bloating, fluid retention, abdominal cramping and breast tenderness; does not increase HDL levels as much as estrogen; blocks vasodilation of the coronary arteries produced by estrogen therapy

menarche: the onset of menstruation

menopause: the cessation of menstruation and the end of fertility; occurs between ages 48 to 52 years; most common symptoms of menopause are hot flashes, urinary disturbances and changes in vaginal tissue; after menopause, estrogen is no longer produced in the ovaries so the adrenal glands compensate for the decline of estrogen production by secreting certain androgens into the bloodstream converted elsewhere in the body (usually fat cells) into estrogen; physiology is unique so menopausal symptoms vary among women

meta-analysis: a statistical analysis of research that pools data from several studies

metacarpal: the part of the hand between the wrist and the fingers

mestranol: a synthetic estrogen used in HRT; a chemical variant of ethinyl estradiol that is also used in oral contraceptives.

metastasis: the proliferation of cancer cells throughout the body by the bloodstream or lymphatic system

methyltestosterone: an androgenic hormone used in HRT

microalbuminuria: a marker of early vascular endothelial damage; defined as urinary albumin excretion of 30 to 300 mg per hour; associated with an increased risk of kidney and cardiovascular disease

micronized progesterone: a natural progesterone; is derived from wild yams or soy beans and is different chemically from commercial progestin frequently prescribed in combination with estrogen; not well absorbed and can be destroyed by stomach or liver enzymes; separated into small particles and encapsulated in oil to prevent breakdown

morbidity: the condition of being diseased; a disease rate

mortality: death

multiparity: having two or more pregnancies that resulted in offspring

natural progesterone: used for the treatment of uterine bleeding, abnormal menstrual cycle and hormone replacement therapy with estrogen (combined therapy) or alone; derived from wild yams or soy beans and prepared in a laboratory (cream or micronized); different chemically from commercial progestins used in HRT

neoplasia: the condition of abnormal cell growth which is uncontrolled and progressive

neoplastic: pertaining to any new or abnormal growth

nonvertebral: not in the spine

norethindrone acetate: a type of progestogen derived from testosterone used in combined therapy

Norgestrel: an androgenic progestogen

nulliparity: never giving birth to a live infant

nulliparous: having never given birth

odds ratio (relative risk estimate): odds of disease in those exposed divided by the odds of the disease in those not exposed; odds of exposure in those who have disease divided by odds of exposure in those who do not have disease; a good approximation of relative risk between exposed and the nonexposed if the disease is rare; used in case-control studies and some cohort studies

oestrogens: European term for estrogen

oophorectomy: surgical removal of the ovaries

osteoporosis: disease of the bones involving demineralization, bone fractures and loss of stature; bone resorption exceeds bone formation; risk increases in aging men (one-third of all hip fractures) and postmenopausal women; risk factors include existing fractures and low bone mineral density, increasing age, gender (women are at greater risk than men), race (Caucasians and Asian women are at higher risk); bone structure and body weight (small boned and lean women are at greater risk), menopausal and menstrual history (early menopause, cessation of menstruation due to anorexia, bulimia or excessive exercise), lifestyle (smoking, alcohol and tobacco consumption, lack of weight-bearing exercise, inadequate calcium intake), medications and disease (corticosteroids, endocrine disorders, rheumatoid arthritis, immobilization)

ovarian adenocarcinomas: malignant ovarian tumors

ovarian cancer: the most common fatal gynecologic malignancy (5-year survival rate of about 25–30 percent percent); heredity plays a role in about 5 percent of all ovarian cancer; two major types of ovarian cancer are epithelial and germ cell; epithelial ovarian cancer the most common form, is typed as serous, mucinous, endometroid, Brenner or clear cell tumors; epithelial tumors are classifed as benign, borderline malignant or malignant; five percent of cases may be genetically related; occurs most often after menopause in the seventh decade; years of ovulation damaging the surface epithelium of the ovary and repeated exposure to estrogen may be the causes of ovarian cancer; obesity, exposure to talcum powder, infertility, nulliparity and infertility drugs have also been associated with the development of ovarian cancer

ovulation: release of the egg from the ovaries occurring monthly during the premenopausal years

PAI-1 (plasminogen-activator inhibitor type 1): an inhibitor of fibrinolysis in humans; increases in women after menopause and may contribute to the risk of cardiovascular disease

Papanicolaou smear: staining procedure for the detection of various conditions malignant and premalignant) for the vagina, cervix and endometrium; cells are obtained by smears, fixed stained and examined microscopically

parity: refers to offspring of a woman

percutaneous: affected or performed through the skin; transdermal

perimenopause: the time before the last menstrual period before menopause; characterized by irregular periods, hot flashes, changes in sleeping patterns, fatigue, heart palpitations, vaginal dryness, mood swings and weight gain; symptoms vary in women

phlebitis: inflammation of a vein

phlebothrombosis: presence of a clot in a vein not associated with inflammation of the wall of the vein

phosphate: a biochemical bone marker

photon absorptiometry (single): measures bone mineral content in the forearm and wrist

plaque: composed of fats that clogs the artery walls; reduce the blood flow through the arteries which can break open and trigger a heart attack or stroke; can become hardened by calcium deposits and result in another condition called arteriosclerosis, hardening of the arteries

plasma: the fluid portion of the blood in which other components are suspended

plasma renin substrate: a sensitive marker of estrogenic action on the liver

plasmin: involved in controlling blood clotting; can dissolve fibrin clots

postmenopause: when a woman has stopped menstruation for a year

prevalence: the number of people in a population who have a disease at a given point in time *prevalence rate:* measure of the total number of cases of a disease at a given time divided by the total population

precursor: a substance from which another substance is formed

Premarin: trade name of an estrogen used in HRT; derived from pregnant mares

progesterone: used for the treatment of uterine bleeding, abnormal menstrual cycle and hormone replacement therapy with estrogen (combined therapy) or alone; derived from wild yams or soy beans and prepared in a laboratory (cream or micronized); different chemically from commercial progestins used in HRT

progestin: name for synthetic progesterone; used in combined therapy with estrogen

progestogens: another name for progestin which is used in combined therapy (estrogen plus progestin) to prevent abnormal endometrial growth

prometrium: a natural micronized progesterone

prophylactic: preventing or guarding against

prospective study (cohort): a study in which data are obtained on health changes of subjects over a given future period; study participants are seleted after the fact according to some criteria and then followed into the future

prothrombotic mutation: a variation in a gene resulted in an increased risk of the development of a thrombus, a blood clot that is stationary or sticks to a vessel wall; can result in a heart attack

Provera: a trade name for a commercial progestin

proximal forearm: forearm closest to body

pulmonary embolism: blood clot in the lungs

quantitative computed tomography: a computerized analysis using x-rays to measure bone mineral density in the spine

radius: bone on the outer or thumb side of the forearm

raloxifene: a synthetic alternative to HRT (estrogen therapy or combined therapy); called a SERM (selective estrogen receptor modulator) because it competes with estrogen at cell-receptor sites; used to treat osteoporosis; unlike estrogen, it may reduce a woman's risk of breast cancer and does not increase the risk of endometrial cancer; negative effects include hot flashes and increased risk of embolism or deep vein thrombosis

random variation: statistical chance

relative hazard: relative risk

relative risk (risk ratio/rate ratio): a ratio of the incidence rate between exposed populations and unexposed population; ratio of two risk factors; risk of the exposed divided by the risk of the unexposed

relative risk estimate: the same as odds ratio; used in case-control studies as a measure of risk

retrospecitve study (case-control): data are collected from a study group in the past; prior exposure is determined in cases and controls

risk: the probability that an indiviudal will develop a disease or experience a change in health over a given time period; probabiltiy of an event occurring over a given time period

selection bias: an error in a study that is a result of the way in which study participants are chosen

selective estrogen receptor modulators (SERMS): e.g., raloxifene, a synthetic alternative to HRT (estrogen therapy or combined therapy); called a selective estrogen receptor modulator because it competes with estrogen at cell-receptor sites *sequential combined therapy:* hormone replacement therapy in which estrogen is given first followed by a shorter duration of progestin plus estrogen

serum calcium: a biochemical marker of bone turnover

single-photon absorptiometry: measures bone mineral content in the forearm and the wrist; measures only cortical bone and not trabecular bone

somatometry: measurement of the body

S-phase: a phase in the cell growth cycle in which DNA synthesis occurs

spurious: false, inaccurate

synthetic estrogens: created in the laboratory; including ethinyl estradiol, estradiol valerate, estriol and other estrogens; degrade slowly in the liver and other tissues

stenosis: narrowing or stricture

stroke (hemorrhagic): a blood vessel to the brain ruptures preventing blood from reaching the brain's tissues

stroke (ischemic stroke): a blood vessel to the brain becomes blocked by either a clot or plaque in the vessel; blood cannot reach the brain tissue beyond the clot

systolic blood pressure: a measure of blood pressure (higher number); stage of the heart beat when the heart contracts and the chambers pump blood

thromboembolic: refers to the condition in which there is an obstruction of a blood vessel usually a blood clot

thromboemobolic disorders: conditions in which there is an obstruction of a blood vessel with a clot originating somewhere else in the bloodstream

thromboembolism: obstruction of a blood vessel with a clot carried by the bloodstream from the site or origin to plug another vessel

thrombophlebitis: inflammation of a vein associated with clot formation

total cholesterol/HDL cholesterol: the ratio of LDL cholesterol to HDL cholesterol; the lower the ratio, the lower the risk of developing heart disease

trabecular: porous, honeycomb inner part of bones

transdermal estrogen: estrogen administered as a patch worn on the skin and changed about twice a week; estradiol enters the bloodstream as estradiol and doesn't have to be processed by the liver, avoiding overstimuation of the liver and unwanted side effects of oral estrogen; may not have the beneficial cardiovascular effects of oral estrogen

triglycerides: a fat synthesized from carbohydrates found in the bloodstream; higher levels may be associated with heart disease

unopposed estrogen: estrogen used alone not in combination with a progestogen

urinary calcium excretion: elevated levels of calcium in the urine are associated with bone loss

urinary incontinence: failure of voluntary control of urination

vasomotor symptoms: menopausal symptoms such as hot flashes and night sweats

venous: of or pertaining to the veins

venous thromboembolism: obstruction of a blood vessel with a clot carried by the blood stream from the site or origin to plug another vessel; embolism in which the clot originates in the veins

very low density lipoprotein (VLDL): carries triglycerides in the bloodstream

zinc excretion: extent of elevated urinary zinc excretion in osteoporotic women; associated with the severity of osteoporosis; a marker of osteoporosis

Bibliography

HRT Research

Adami H-O et al. Risk of cancer in women receiving hormone replacement therapy. *International Journal of Cancer*, November 1989; 44:833–839.

Aloia J et al. Calcium supplementation with and without hormone replacement therapy to prevent postmenopausal bone loss. *Annals of Internal Medicine*, January 1994; 120:97–102.

Annegers J et al. Ovarian cancer, incidence and case-control study. *Cancer*, February 1979; 43:723–729.

Antunes C et al. Endometrial cancer and estrogen use. *The New England Journal of Medicine*, January 1979; 300:9–13.

Baron Y, Galea R, and Brincat M. Carotid artery wall changes in estrogen-treated and -untreated postmenopausal women. *Obstetrics and Gynecology*, June 1998; 91: 982–985.

Barrett-Connor E and Kritz-Silverstein D. Estrogen replacement therapy and cognitive function in older women. *Journal of the American Medical Association*, May 1993; 269:2637–2641.

Beresford S et al. Risk of endometrial cancer in relation to use of oestrogen combined with cyclic progestagen therapy in postmenopausal women. *Lancet*, February 1997; 349:458–461.

Bergkvist L et al. Risk factors for breast and endometrial cancer in a cohort of women treated with menopausal oestrogen. *International Journal of Epidemiology*, December 1988; 17: 732–737.

Bergkvist L et al. The risk of breast cancer after estrogen and estrogen-progestin replacement. *The New England Journal of Medicine*, August 1989; 321:293–297.

Bland K et al. The effects of exogenous estrogen replacement therapy of the breast cancer risk and mammographic parenchymal pattern. *Cancer*, June 1980; 45: 3027–3033.

Boston Collaborative Drug Surveillance Program. Surgically confirmed gallbladder disease, venous thromoembolism and breast tumors in relation to postmenopausal estrogen therapy. *New England Journal of Medicine*, January 1974; 290:15–19.

247

Brenner D et al. Postmenopausal estrogen replacement therapy and the risk of Alzheimer's disease: a population-based case-control study. *American Journal of Epidemiology*, August 1994; 140:262–267.

Brinton L et al. Menopausal estrogens use and risk of breast cancer. *Cancer*, May 1981; 47:2517–2522.

Bruschi F et al. Lipoprotein (a) and other lipids after oophorectomy and estrogen replacement therapy. *Obstetrics and Gynecology*, December 1996; 88:950–954.

Burch J and Byrd B. Effects of long-term administration of estrogen on the occurrence of mammary cancer in women. *Annals of Surgery*, September 1971; 174:414–418.

Burch J, Byrd B, and Vaughn W. The effects of long-term estrogen on hysterectomized women. *American Journal of Obstetrics and Gynecology*, March 1974; 118:778–782.

Buring J et al. A prospective cohort study of postmenopausal women hormone use and risk of breast cancer in US women. *American Journal of Epidemiology*, June 1987; 125:939–947.

Bush T et al. Cardiovascular mortality and noncontraceptive use of estrogen in women: results from the lipid research clinics program follow-up study. *Circulation*, June 1987; 75:1102–1109.

Byrd B, Burch J, and Vaughn W. The impact of long term estrogen support after hysterectomy. *The Annals of Surgery*, May 1977; 185:574–580.

Calle E et al. Estrogen replacement therapy and risk of fatal colon cancer in a April 1995; 87:517–523.

Cauley J et al. Bone mineral density and risk of breast cancer in older women: the study of osteoporotic fractures. *Journal of the American Medical Association*, November 1996; 276:1401–1406.

Chen C-L et al. Hormone replacement therapy in relation to breast cancer. *Journal of the American Medical Association*, February 2002; 287:734–741.

Christ M, Seyffart K, and Wehling M. Attenuation of heart-rate variability in postmenopausal women on progestin-containing hormone replacement therapy (Research Letters). *The Lancet*, June 1999; 353:1939–1940.

Christiansen C, Christensen M, and Transbøl I. Bone mass in postmenopausal women after withdrawal of oestrogen/gestagen replacement therapy. *The Lancet*, February 1981; 1:459–461.

Clisham P et al. Long-term transdermal estradiol therapy: effects on endometrial histology and bleeding patterns. *Obstetrics and Gynecology*, February 1992; 79:196–201.

Cobleigh M et al. Hormone replacement therapy and high S phase in breast cancer. *Journal of the American Medical Association*, April 1999; 281:1528–1530.

Col N et al. Individualizing therapy to prevent long-term consequences of estrogen deficiency in postmenopausal women. *Archives of Internal Medicine*, July 1999; 159:1458–1466.

Colditz G, Egan K, and Stampfer M. Hormone replacement therapy and risk of breast cancer: results from epidemiologic studies. *American Journal of Obstetrics and Gynecology*, May 1993; 168:1473–1479.

Colditz G et al. Prospective study of estrogen replacement therapy and risk of breast cancer in postmenopausal women. *Journal of the American Medical Association*, November 1990; 264:2648–2652.

Colditz G et al. The use of estrogens and progestins and the risk of breast cancer. *The New England Journal of Medicine*, June 1995; 332:1589–1593.

Connor E and Silverstein D. Estrogen replacement therapy and cognitive function in older women. *Journal of the American Medical Association*, May 1993; 269: 2637–2641.

Cramer D et al. Determinants of ovarian cancer risk. I. Reproductive experiences and family history. *Journal of the National Cancer Institute*, October 1983; 71:711–716.

Cummings S et al. The effect of raloxifene on risk of breast cancer in postmenopausal women: results from the MORE randomized trial. *Journal of the American Medical Association*, June 1999; 281:2189–2197.

Cummings S et al. Endogenous hormones and the risk of hip and vertebral fractures among older women. *The New England Journal of Medicine*, September 1998; 339:733–738.

Cummings S et al. Serum estradiol level and risk of breast cancer during treatment with raloxifene. *Journal of the American Medical Association*, January 2002; 287: 216–220.

Daly E et al. Risk of venous thromboembolism in users of hormone replacement therapy. *The Lancet*, October 1996; 348:977–980.

Davies G et al. Adverse events reported by postmenopausal women in controlled trials with raloxifene. *Obstetrics and Gynecology*, April 1999; 93:558–565.

Derby C et al. Prior and current health characteristics of postmenopausal estrogen replacement therapy users compared with nonusers. *The American Journal of Obstetrics and Gynecology*, August 1995; 173:544–550.

DiSaia P et al. Hormone replacement therapy in breast cancer survivors: a cohort study. *American Journal of Obstetrics and Gynecology*, May 1996; 174:1494–1498.

Eeles R et al. Hormone replacement therapy and survival after surgery for ovarian cancer. *British Medical Journal*, February 1991; 302:259–262.

Espeland M et al. Estrogen replacement therapy and progression of intimal-medial thickness in the carotid arteries of postmenopausal women. *American Journal of Epidemiology*, November 1995; 142:1011–1019.

Ettinger B, Genant H, and Cann C. Long-term estrogen replacement therapy prevents bone loss and fractures. *Annals of Internal Medicine*, March 1985; 102:319–324.

Ettinger B, Genant H, and Cann C. Postmenopausal bone loss is prevented by treatment with low-dosage estrogen with calcium. *Annals of Internal Medicine*, January 1987; 106:40–45.

Ettinger B et al. Comparison of endometrial growth produced by unopposed conjugated estrogens or by micronized estradiol in postmenopausal women. *American Journal of Obstetrics and Gynecology*, January 1997; 176:112–117.

Ettinger B et al. Reduced mortality associated with long-term postmenopausal estrogen therapy. *Obstetrics and Gynecology*, January 1996; 87:6–12.

Ettinger B et al. Reduction of vertebral fracture risk in postmenopausal women with osteoporosis treated with raloxifene: results from a 3-year randomized clinical trial. *Journal of the American Medical Association*, August 1999; 282:637–645.

Ewertz M. Influence of non-contraceptive exogenous and endogenous sex hormones on breast cancer in Denmark. *The International Journal of Cancer*, December 1988; 42:832–838.

Fantl J et al. Efficacy of estrogen supplementation in the treatment of urinary incontinence. *Obstetrics and Gynecology*, November 1996; 88:745–749.

Felson D et al. The effects of postmenopausal estrogen therapy of bone density in elderly women. *The New England Journal of Medicine*, October 1993; 329:1141–1146.

Gallagher J and Kable W. Effect of progestin therapy on cortical and trabecular bone: comparison with estrogen. *The American Journal of Medicine*, February 1991; 90:171–177.

Gambrell R, Maier R, and Sanders B. Decreased incidence of breast cancer in postmenopausal estrogen-progestogen users. *Obstetrics and Gynecology*, Oct.–Dec. 1983; 62:435–443.

Gambrell R et al. Decreased incidence of breast cancer in postmenopausal estrogen-progestogen users. *Obstetrics and Gynecology*, Oct.–Dec.1983; 62:435–443.

Gapstur S, Morrow M, and Sellers T. Hormone replacement therapy and risk breast cancer with a favorable histology, results of the Iowa Women's Health Study. *Journal of the American Medical Association*, June 1999; 281:2091–2097.

Garg P et al. Hormone replacement therapy and the risk of epithelial ovarian carcinoma: a meta-analysis. *Obstetrics and Gynecology*, September 1998; 92:472–479.

Gelfand M and Ferenczy A. A prospective 1-year study of estrogen and progestin in postmenopausal women: effects on the endometrium. *Obstetrics and Gynecology*, September 1989; 74:398–401.

Genant H et al. Effect of estrone sulfate on postmenopausal bone loss. *Obstetrics and Gynecology*, October 1990; 76:579–584.

Genant H et al. Low-dose esterified estrogen therapy: effects on bone, plasma estradiol concentrations, endometrium, and lipid levels. *Archives of Internal Medicine*, December 1997; 157:2609–2615.

Gilabert J et al. The effect of estrogen replacement therapy with or without progestogen on the fibrinolytic system and coagulation inhibitors in postmenopausal status. *American Journal of Obstetrics and Gynecology*, December 1995; 173:1849–1854.

Grady D et al. Cardiovascular disease outcomes during 6.8 years of hormone therapy: Heart and Estrogen/Progestin Replacement Study Follow-up (HERS II). *Journal of the American Medical Association*, July 2002; 288:49–57.

Grady D et al. Hormone replacement therapy and endometrial cancer risk: a meta-analysis. *Obstetrics and Gynecology*, February 1995; 85:304–313.

Gray L, Christopherson W, and Hoover R. Estrogens and endometrial carcinoma. *Obstetrics and Gynecology*, April 1977; 49:385–389.

Greendale G et al. Symptom relief and side effects of postmenopausal hormones: results from the postmenopausal estrogen/progestin intervention trial. *Obstetrics and Gynecology*, December 1998; 92:982–988.

Grey A et al. Effect of hormone replacement therapy on bone mineral density in postmenopausal women with mild primary hyperparathyroidism. *Annals of Internal Medicine*, September 1996; 125:360–367.

Grodstein F et al. Postmenopausal estrogen and progestin use and the risk of cardiovascular disease. *The New England Journal of Medicine*, August 1996; 35:453–461.

Grodstein F et al. Postmenopausal hormone therapy and mortality. *The New England Journal of Medicine*, June 1997; 336:1769–1775.

Grodstein F et al. Prospective study of exogenous hormones and risk of pulmonary embolism in women. *Lancet*, October 1996; 348:983–987.

Gruchow H et al. Postmenopausal use of estrogen and occlusion of coronary arteries. *American Heart Journal*, May 1988; 115:954–962.

Gutthann S et al. Hormone replacement therapy and risk of venous thromboembolism: population based case-control study. *British Medical Journal*, March 1997; 314:796–800.

Haines C et al. Effect of oral estradiol on Lp(a) and other lipoproteins in postmenopausal women. *Archives of Internal Medicine*, April 1996; 156:866–872.

Hammond C et al. Effects of long-term estrogen replacement therapy: II Neoplasia. *American Journal of Obstetrics and Gynecology*, March 1979; 133:537–546.

Harris R et al. Characteristics relating to ovarian cancer risk: Collaborative analysis of 12 US case-control studies (Part II: Epithelial tumors of low malignant potential in white women). *American Journal of Epidemiology*, November 1992; 136:1204–1211.

Harris S et al. The effects of estrone (Ogen) on spinal bone density of postmenopausal women. *Archives of Internal Medicine*, October 1991; 151:1980–1984.

Hartge P et al. Menopause and ovarian cancer. *American Journal of Epidemiology*, May 1988; 127:990–998.

Haskell S, Richardson E, and Horwitz R. The effect of estrogen replacement therapy on cognitive function in women: a critical review of the literature. *Journal of Clinical Epidemiology*, November 1997; 50:1249–1264.

Hassager C et al. The long-term effect of oral and percutaneous estradiol on plasma renin substrate and blood pressure. *Circulation*, October 1987; 76:753–758.

Heckbert S et al. Risk of recurrent coronary events in relation to use and recent initiation of postmenopausal hormone therapy. *Archives of Internal Medicine*, July 2001; 161:1709–1713.

Hemminki E and McPherson K. Impact of postmenopausal hormone therapy on cardiovascular events and cancer, pooled data from clinical trials. *British Medical Journal*, July 1997; 315:149–153.

Henderson B, Paganini-Hill A, and Ross R. Decreased mortality in users of estrogen replacement therapy. *Archives of Internal Medicine*, January 1991; 151:75–78.

Herzberg M et al. The effect of estrogen replacement therapy on zinc in serum and urine. *Obstetrics and Gynecology*, June 1996; 87:1035–1039.

Hiatt R et al. Exogenous estrogens and breast cancer after bilateral oophorectomy. *Cancer*, July 1984; 54:139–144.

Hildreth N et al. An epidemiologic study of epithelial carcinoma of the ovary. *American Journal of Epidemiology*, September 1981; 114:398–405.

Hlatky M et al. Quality-of-life and depressive symptoms in postmenopausal women after receiving hormone therapy (results from the Heart and Estrogen/Progestin Replacement Study Trial. *Journal of the American Medical Association*, February 2002; 287:591–597.

Hoover R et al. Menopausal estrogens and breast cancer. *The New England Journal of Medicine*, August 1976; 295:401–405.

Horsman A et al. The effect of estrogen dose on postmenopausal bone loss. *The New England Journal of Medicine*, December 1983; 309:1405–1407.

Horsman A et al. Prospective trial of oestrogen and calcium in postmenopausal women. *British Medical Journal*, September 1977; 2:789–792.

Horwitz R and Steward K. Effects of clinical features on the association of estrogens and breast cancer. *The American Journal of Medicine*, February 1984; 76:192–198.

Hulka B et al. Estrogen and endometrial cancer: cases and two control groups form North Carolina. *American Journal of Obstetrics and Gynecology*, May 1980; 137:92–101.

Hulley S et al. Noncardiovascular disease outcomes during 6.8 years of hormone therapy: Heart and Estrogen/Progestin Replacement Study Follow-up (HERS II). *Journal of the American Medical Association*, July 2002; 288:58–66.

Hulley S et al. Randomized trial of estrogen plus progestin for secondary prevention of coronary heart disease in postmenopausal women. *Journal of the American Medical Association*, August 1998; 280:605–613.

Hunt K et al. Long-term surveillance of mortality and cancer incidence in women receiving hormone replacement therapy. *The British Journal of Obstetrics and Gynecology*, July 1987; 94:620–635.

Hutchinson T, Polansky S, and Feinstein A. Postmenopausal estrogens protect against fractures of hip and distal radius. *The Lancet*, October 1979; 2:705–709.

Jelovsek F et al. Risk of exogenous estrogen therapy and endometrial cancer. *American Journal of Obstetrics and Gynecology*, May 1980; 137:85–90.

Jick H et al. Replacement estrogens and breast cancer. *American Journal of Epidemiology*, November 1980; 112:586–594.

Jick H et al. Replacement estrogens and endometrial cancer. *The New England Journal of Medicine*, February 1979; 300:218–222.

Jick H et al. Risk of hospital admission for idiopathic venous thromboembolism among users of postmenopausal oestrogens. *The Lancet*, October 1996; 348:981–983.

Kampen D and Sherwin B. Estrogen use and verbal memory in healthy postmenopausal women. *Obstetrics and Gynecology*, June 1994; 83:979–983.

Kaufman D et al. Estrogen replacement therapy and the risk of breast cancer: results from case-control surveillance study. *The American Journal of Epidemiology*, May 1991; 134:1375–1385.

Kaufman D et al. Noncontraceptive estrogen use and epithelial ovarian cancer. *American Journal of Epidemiology*, December 1989; 130:1142–1151.

Kaufman D et al. Noncontraceptive estrogen use and the risk of breast cancer. *Journal of the American Medical Association*, July 1984; 252:63–77.

Kim C et al. Changes in Lp(a) lipoprotein and lipid levels after cessation of female sex hormone production and estrogen replacement therapy. *Archives of Internal Medicine*, March 1996; 156:500–504.

Koh K et al. Effects of hormone-replacement therapy on fibrinolysis in postmenopausal women. *The New England Journal of Medicine*, March 1997; 336:683–689.

Kohrt W, Ehsani A, and Birge S. HRT preserves increases in bone mineral density and reduction in body fat after a supervised exercise program. *Applied Physiology*, January 1998; 84:1506–1512.

Komulainen M et al. Prevention of femoral and lumber bone loss with hormone replacement therapy and vitamin D-3 in early postmenopausal women: a population-based 5-year randomized trial. *Journal of Clinical Endocrinology and Metabolism*, 1999; 84:546–552.

Kritz-Silverstein D and Barrett-Connor E. Long-term postmenopausal hormone use, obesity, and fat distribution in older women. *Journal of the American Medical Association*, January 1996; 275:46–49.

Lacey J et al. Menopausal hormone replacement therapy and risk of ovarian cancer. *Journal of the American Medical Association*, July 2002; 288:334–341.

LaVecchia C et al. Non-contraceptive oestrogens and the risk of breast cancer in women. *International Journal of Cancer*, December 1986; 38:853–858.

Lawson D et al. Exogenous estrogens and breast cancer. *American Journal of Epidemiology*, November 1981; 114:710–713.

Laya M et al. Effects of estrogen replacement of the specificity and sensitivity of screening mammography. *Journal of the National Cancer Institute*, May 1996; 88: 643–649.

LeBlanc E et al. Hormone replacement therapy and cognition. *Journal of the American Medical Association*, March 2001; 285:1489–1499.

Lindsay R, Hart D, and Lark M. The minimum effective dose of estrogen for prevention of postmenopausal bone loss. *Obstetrics and Gynecology*, June 1984; 63: 759–763.

Lindsay R et al. Bone response to termination of oestrogen treatment.*The Lancet*, June 1978; 1:1325–1327.

Lindsay R et al. Effect of lower doses of conjugated equine estrogens with and without medroxyprogesterone acetate on bone in early postmenopausal women. *Journal of the American Medical Association*, May 2002; 287:2668–2676.

Lindsay R et al. Long-term prevention of postmenopausal osteoporosis by oestrogen.*The Lancet*, May 1976; 1:1038–1040.

Lipworth L et al. Oral contraceptives, menopausal estrogens, and the risk of breast cancer a case-control study in Greece. *The International Journal of Cancer*, September 1995; 62:548–551.

Mack T et al. Estrogens and endometrial cancer in a retirement community. *The New England Journal of Medicine*, June 1976; 294:1262–1267.

Manolio T et al. Association of postmenopausal estrogen use with cardiovascular disease and its risk factors in older women. *Circulation*, November 1993; 88:2163–2171.

Marslew U et al. Two new combinations of estrogen and progestogen for prevention of post-menopausal bone loss: long-term effects on bone, calcium and lipid metabolism, climacteric symptoms and bleeding. *Obstetrics and Gynecology*, February 1992; 79:202–210.

McDonald T et al. Exogenous estrogen and endometrial carcinoma: case-control and incidence study. *American Journal of Obstetrics and Gynecology*, March 1977; 127:572–579.

Medical Research Council's General Practice Research Framework. Randomized comparison of oestrogen versus oestrogen plus progestogen hormone replacement therapy in women with hysterectomy. *British Medical Journal*, February 1996; 312:473–477.

Michaëlsson K et al. Hormone replacement therapy and risk of hip fracture: population based case-control study. *British Medical Journal*, June 1998; 316:1858–1862.

Mills P et al. Prospective study of exogenous hormone use and breast cancer in a Seventh-day Adventist. *Cancer*, August 1989; 64:591–597.

Monster T et al. Oral contraceptive use and hormone replacement therapy are associated with microalbuminuria. *Archives of Internal Medicine*, September 2001; 161:2000–2005.

Mulnard R et al. Estrogen replacement therapy for treatment of mild to moderate alzheimer disease. *Journal of the American Medical Association*, February 2001; 283: 1007–1015.

Munk-Jensen N et al. Continuous combined and sequential estradiol and norethindrone acetate treatment of postmenopausal women. Effect on plasma lipoproteins in a two-year placebo-controlled trial. *American Journal of Obstetrics and Gynecology*, July 1994; 171:132–138.

Nabulski A et al. Association of hormone-replacement with various cardiovascular risk factors in postmenopausal women. *The New England Journal of Medicine*, April 1993; 328:1069–1075.

Nachtigall L, Nachtigall R, and Beckman R. Estrogen replacement therapy II: a prospective study in the relationship to carcinoma and cardiovascular and metabolic problems.*Obstetrics and Gynecology*, July 1979; 54:74–79.

Naessen T, Berglund L, and Ulmsten U. Bone loss in elderly women prevented by ultralow doses of parenteral 17ß-estradiol. *The American Journal of Obstetrics and Gynecology*, July 1997; 177:115–119.

Newcomb P et al. Long-term hormone replacement therapy and the risk of breast cancer in postmenopausal women. *The American Journal of Epidemiology*, October 1995; 142:788–795.

Nomura A et al. The association of replacement estrogens with breast cancer. *International Journal of Cancer*, January 1986; 37:49–53.

Ottosson U, Johansson B, and Von Schoultz B. Subfractions of high-density lipoprotein cholesterol during estrogen replacement therapy: a comparison between progestogens and natural progesterone. *The American Journal of Obstetrics and Gynecology*, March 1985; 151:746–750.

Paganini-Hill A. The benefits of estrogen replacement therapy on oral health. *Archives of Internal Medicine*, November 1995; 155:2325–2329.

Palmer J et al. Breast cancer risk after estrogen replacement therapy: results from the Toronto Breast Cancer Study. *The American Journal of Epidemiology*, December 1991; 134:1386–1395.

Parazzinni F et al. Case-control study of oestrogen replacement therapy and risk of cervical cancer, *British Medical Journal*, July 1997; 315:85–87.

Paterson M et al. Endometrial disease after treatment with oestrogens and progetogens in the climacteric. *British Medical Journal*, March 1980; 280:822–824.

Perrone G et al. Effect of oral and transdermal hormone replacement therapy on lipid profile and LP(a) level in menopausal women with hypercholesterolemia. *International Journal of Fertility*, Nov.–Dec.1996; 41(6):509–515.

Polo-Kantola P et al. The effect of short-term estrogen replacement therapy on cognition: a randomized, double-blind, cross-over trial in postmenopausal women. *Obstetrics and Gynecology*, March 1998; 91:459–466.

Polychronopoulou A et al. Reproductive variables, tobacco, ethanol, coffee and somatometry as risk factors for ovarian cancer. *International Journal of Cancer*, September 1993; 55:402–407.

Pradhan A et al. Inflammatory biomarkers, hormone replacemnt therapy, and incident coronary heart disease: prospective analysis from the Women's Health Initiative observational study. *Journal of the American Medical Association*, August 2002; 288:980–987.

Prince R et al. Prevention of postmenopausal osteoporosis, a comparative study of exercise, calcium supplementation and hormone-replacement therapy. *The New England Journal of Medicine*, October 1991; 325:1189–1195.

Psaty B et al. Hormone replacement therapy, prothrombotic mutations, and the risk of incident nonfatal myocardial infarction in postmenopausal women. *Journal of the American Medical Association*, February 2001; 285:906–913.

Purdie D et al. Reproductive and other factors and risk of epithelial ovarian cancer: an Australian case-control study. *International Journal of Cancer*, September 1995; 62:678–684.

Raz R and Stamm W. A controlled trial of intravaginal estriol in postmenopausal women with recurrent urinary tract infection. *The New England Journal of Medicine*, September 1993; 329:753–756.

Recker R, Saville P, Heaney R. Effects of estrogens and calcium carbonate on bone loss in postmenopausal women. *Annals of Internal Medicine*, December 1977; 87: 649–654.

Riis B, Thomsen K, and Christiansen C. Does calcium supplementation prevent postmenopausal bone loss? *The New England Journal of Medicine*, January 1987; 316:173–177.

Rodriguez C et al. Estrogen replacement therapy and fatal ovarian cancer. *American Journal Epidemiology*, May 1995; 141:828–835.

Rodriguez C et al. Estrogen replacement therapy and ovarian cancer mortality in a large prospective study of US women. *Journal of the American Medical Association*, March 2001; 285:1460–1465.

Ross R et al. A case-control study of menopausal estrogen therapy and breast cancer. *Journal of the American Medical Association*, April 1980; 243:1635–1639.

Rutter C et al. Changes in breast density associated with initiation, discontinuation, and continuing use of hormone replacement therapy. *Journal of the American Medical Association*, January 2001; 285:171–176.

Sanches-Guerrero J et al. Postmenopausal estrogen therapy and the risk for developing systemic lupus erythematosus. *Annals of Internal Medicine*, March 1995; 122:430–433.

Schairer C et al. Menopausal estrogen and estrogen-progestin replacement therapy and breast cancer risk. *Journal of the American Medical Association*, January 2000; 283:485–491.

Schaumber D st al. Hormone replacement and dry eye syndrome. *Journal of the American Medical Association*, November 2001; 286:2114–2119.

Seeley D et al. Is postmenopausal estrogen therapy associated with neuromuscular functions or falling in elderly women. *Archives of Internal Medicine*, February 1995; 155:293–299.

Selby P and Peacock M. Dose dependent response of symptoms, pituitary, and bone to transdermal oestrogen in postmenopausal women. *British Medical Journal*, November 1986; 293:1337–1339.

Shapiro S et al. Recent and past use of conjugated estrogens in relation to adenocarcinoma of the endometrium. *The New England Journal of Medicine*, August 1980; 303:485–489.

Shaywitz S et al. Effects of estrogen on brain activation patterns in postmenopausal women during working memory tasks. *Journal of the American Medical Association*, April 1999; 281:1197–1202.

Shemesh J et al. Does hormone replacement therapy inhibit coronary artery calcification? *Obstetrics and Gynecology*, June 1997; 89:989–992.

Sherman B, Wallace R, and Bean J. Estrogen use and breast cancer: interaction with body mass. *Cancer*, April 1983; 51:1527–1531.

Shu X et al. Population-based case-control study of ovarian cancer in Shanghai. *Cancer Research*, July 1989; 49:3670–3674.

Smith D et al. Association of exogenous estrogen and endometrial carcinoma. *The New England Journal of Medicine*, December 1975; 293:1164–1166.

Snabes M et al. In normal postmenopausal women physiologic estrogen replacement therapy fails to improve exercise tolerance: A randomized, double-blind, placebo-controlled, crossover trial. *American Journal of Obstetrics and Gynecology,* July 1996; 175:110–113.

Snabes M et al. Physiologic estradiol replacement therapy and cardiac structure and function in normal postmenopausal women: a randomized, double-blind, placebo-controlled, crossover trial. *Obstetrics and Gynecology,* March 1997; 89: 332–339.

Speroff L et al. The comparative effect on bone density, endometrium, and lipids of continuous hormones as replacement therapy (Chart Study). *Journal of American Medical Association,* November 1996; 276:1397–1403.

Stanford J et al. Combined estrogen and progestin hormone replacement therapy in relation to risk of breast cancer in middle age women. *The Journal of the American Medical Association,* July 1995; 274:137–142.

Steinberg K et al. A meta-analysis of the effect of estrogen replacement therapy on the risk of breast cancer. *The Journal of the American Medical Association,* April 1991; 265:1985–1990.

Szklo M et al. Estrogen replacement therapy and cognitive functioning in the atherosclerosis risk in communities (ARIC) study. *American Journal of Epidemiology,* December 1996; 144:1048–1056.

Torgerson D and Bell-Syer S. Hormone replacement therapy and prevention of nonvertebral fractures. *Journal of the American Medical Association,* June 2001; 285:2891–2897.

Villareal D et al. Bone mineral density response to estrogen replacement in frail elderly women. *Journal of the American Medical Association,* August 2001; 286: 815–820.

Wakatsuke A et al. Effect of estrogen and simvastatin on low-density lipoprotein subclasses in hypercholesterolemic postmenopausal women. *Obstetrics and Gynecology,* September 1998; 92:367–372.

Walsh B et al. Effects of postmenopausal estrogen replacement on the concentrations and metabolism of plasma lipoproteins. *The New England Journal of Medicine,* October 1991; 325:1196–1204.

Walsh B et al. Effects of raloxifene on serum and lipids and coagulation factors in healthy postmenopausal women. *Journal of the American Medical Association,* May 1998; 279:1445–1451.

Waters D et al. Effects of hormone replacement therapy and antioxidant vitamin supplements on coronary atherosclerosis in postmenopausal women. *Journal of the American Medical Association,* November 2002; 288:2432–2440.

Weinstein L, Bewtra C, and Gallagher J. Evaluation of a continuous combined low-dose regimen of estrogen-progestin for treatment of the menopausal patient. *American Journal of Obstetrics and Gynecology,* June 1990; 162:1534–1542.

Weiss N. Endometrial cancer in relation to patterns of menopausal estrogen use. *Journal of the American Medical Association,* July 1979; 242:261–264.

Weiss N, Daling J, and Chow W. Incidence of cancer of the large bowel in women in relation to reproductive and hormonal factors. *Journal of the National Cancer Institute,* July 1981; 67:57–60.

Weiss N et al. Decreased risk of fractures of the hip and lower forearm with postmenopausal use of estrogen. *The New England Journal of Medicine,* November 1980; 303:1195–1198.

Weiss N et al. Noncontraceptive estrogen use and the occurrence of ovarian cancer. *Journal of the National Cancer Institute,* January 1982; 68:95–98.

Whittemore A et al. Characteristics relating to ovarian cancer risk: collaborative analysis of 12 U.S. case-control studies (Part I: Invasive epithelial ovarian cancers in white women). *American Journal of Epidemiology*, November 1992; 136:1184–1203.

Whittemore A et al. Personal characteristics relating to risk of invasive epithelial ovarian cancer in older women in the United States. *Cancer*, January 1993; 71:558–565.

Wilson P, Garrison R, and Castelli W. Postmenopausal estrogen use, cigarette smoking and cardiovascular morbidity in women over 50 (The Framingham Study). *The New England Journal of Medicine*, October 1985; 313:1038–1043.

Wimalawansa S et al. A four-year randomized controlled trial of hormone replacement and bisphosphonate, alone or in combination, in women with postmenopausal osteoporosis. *American Journal of Medicine*, March 1998; 104:219–226.

Wingo P et al. The risk of breast cancer in postmenopausal women who have used estrogen replacement therapy. *The Journal of the American Medical Association*, January 1987; 257:209–215.

Woodruff J and Pickar J. Incidence of endometrial hyperplasia in postmenopausal women taking conjugated estrogens (Premarin) with medroxyprogesterone acetate or conjugated estrogens alone. *American Journal of Obstetrics and Gynecology*, May 1994; 170:1213–1223.

Writing Group for the PEPI Trial. Effects of estrogen or estrogen/progestin regimens on heart disease risk factor in postmenopausal women: the postmenopausal estrogen/progestin interventions (PEPI) trial. *Journal of the American Medical Association*, January 1995; 273:199–208.

Writing Group for the PEPI Trial. Effects of hormone replacement therapy on endometrial histology in postmenopausal women. *Journal of the American Medical Association*, February 1996; 275:370–375.

Writing Group for the PEPI Trial. Effects of hormone therapy on bone mineral density: Results from the postmenopausal estrogen/progestin intervention (PEPI) trial. *Journal of the American Medical Association*, November 1996; 276: 1389–1396.

Writing Group for the Women's Health Initiative Investigators. Risks and benefits of estrogen plus progestin in healthy postmenopausal women: principal results from the Women's Health Initiative randomized controlled trial. *Journal of the American Medical Association*; July 2002; 288:321–333.

Yaffe K et al. Estrogen therapy in postmenopausal women: effects on cognitive function and dementia. *Journal of the American Medical Association*, March 1998; 279:688–695.

Zandi P et al. Hormone replacement therapy and incidence of alzheimer disease in older women (The Cache County Study). *Journal of the American Medical Association*, November 2002; 288:2123–2129.

Ziel H and Finkle W. Association of estrone with the development of endometrial carcinoma. *American Journal of Obstetrics and Gynecology*, April 1976; 124:735–739.

Ziel H and Finkle W. Increased risk of endometrial carcinoma among users of conjugated estrogens. *The New England Journal of Medicine*, December 1975; 293:1167–1170.

Additional Sources

Abramson J. *Making Sense of Data.* New York: Oxford University Press, 1988.

Alexandersen P et al. Ipriflavone in the treatment of postmenopausal osteoporosis: a randomized controlled trial. *Journal of the American Medical Association,* March 2001; 285:1482–1488.

ALLHAT Collaborative Research Group. Major outcomes in high-risk hypertensive patients randomized to angiotensin-converting enzyme inhibitor or calcium channel blocker vs diuretic (The Antihypertensive and Lipid-Lowering Treatment to Prevent Heart Attack Trial). *Journal of the American Medical Association,* December 2002; 288:2981–2997.

Anderson J et al. Meta-analysis of the effects of soy protein intake on serum lipids. *The New England Journal of Medicine,* August 1995; 333:276–282.

Arnot B. *The Breast Cancer Prevention Diet.* Boston: Little Brown and Company, 1998.

Ascherio A et al. Prospective study of nutritional factors, blood pressure, and hypertension among US women. *Hypertension,* May 1996; 27:1065–1072.

Ascherio A et al. Trans-fatty intake and risk of myocardial infarction. *Circulation,* January 1994; 89:94–101.

Atalay M and Sen C. Physical exercise and antioxidant defenses in the heart. *Annals of the New York Academy of Sciences,* June 1999; 874:169–177.

Ballantyne C. Low-density lipoproteins and risk for coronary artery disease. *American Journal of Cardiology,* November 1998; 82:3Q–12Q.

Barnett P et al. Psychological stress and the progression of carotid artery disease. *Journal of Hypertension,* January 1997; 15:49–55.

Blankenhorn D et al. The influence of diet on the appearance of new lesions in human coronary arteries. *Journal of the American Medical Association,* March 1990; 263:1646–1652.

Blot W. Invited commentary: more evidence of increased risks of cancer among alcohol drinkers. *American Journal of Epidemiology,* December 1999; 150:1138–1140.

Brandi M et al. New strategies: ipriflavone, strontium, vitamin D metabolites and analogs. *American Journal of Medicine,* November 1993; 95:69S–74S.

Brattström L et al. (Homocysteine Lowering Trialists'Collaboration). Lowering blood homocysteine with folic acid based supplements: meta-analysis of randomised trials. *British Medical Journal,* March 1998; 316:894–898.

Cashin-Hemphill L and Vailas L. Hormone-replacement therapy compared with Simvastatin for postmenopausal women with hypercholesterolemia. To the Editor. *New England Journal of Medicine,* January 1998; 338:63.

Cashin-Hemphill L et al. Beneficial effects of colestipol-niacin on coronary atherosclerosis. a 4-year follow-up. *Journal of the American Medical Association,* December 1990; 264:3013–3017.

Castelli W. Cholesterol and lipids in the risk of coronary artery disease—The Framingham Heart Study. *Canadian Journal of Cardiology,* July 1988; Supplement A: 5A–10A.

Cauley J et al. The epidemiology of serum sex hormones in postmenopausal women. *American Journal of Epidemiology,* June 1989; 129:1120–1131.

Chan K et al. Inhibitors of hydroxmethylglutaryl-coenzyme A reductase and risk of fracture among older women. *Lancet,* June 2000; 335:2185–2188.

Chen Z et al. Indications for early aspirin use in acute ischemic stroke: a combined analysis of 40,000 radomized patients from the Chinese Acute Stroke Trial and International Stroke Trial. *Stroke,* June 2000; 31:1240–1249.

Clarke R et al. Dietary lipids and blood cholesterol: a quantitative meta-analysis of metabolic ward studies. *British Medical Journal,* January 1997; 314:112–117.

Cohn V. *New and Numbers.* Ames: Iowa State University Press, 1989.

Conney S. *The Menopause Industry.* Alameda: Hunter House, 1994.

Cummings H and Bingham S. Diet and the prevention of cancer. *British Medical Journal,* December 1998; 317:1636–1640.

Daly L and Bourke G. *Interpretation and Uses of Medical Statistics.* Malden: Blackwell Science, 2000.

Daniels S et al. *Medical Epidemiology.* Ed. Raymond S. Greenberg, MD, PhD. Norwalk: Appleton & Lange, 1993.

Darling G et al. Estrogen and progestin compared with simvastatin for hypercholesterolemia in postmenopausal women. *New England Journal of Medicine,* August 1997; 337:595–601.

Detre K et al. Secondary prevention and lipid lowering: results and implications. *American Heart Journal,* November 1985; 110:1123–1127.

Dollinger M, Rosenbaum E and Cable G. *Everyone's Guide to Cancer Therapy.* Kansas City: Universal Press Syndicate Co., 1994.

Fairfield K and Fletcher R. Vitamins for chronic disease prevention in adults. *Journal of the American Medical Association,* June 2002; 287:3116–3126.

Fleischauer A et al. Dietary antioxidants, supplements, and risk of epithelial ovarian cancer. *Nutrition and Cancer,* 2001; 40:92–98.

Franceschini G et al. Omega-3 fatty acids selectively raise high-density lipoprotein levels in healthy volunteers. *Metabolism,* December 1991; 40:1283–1286.

Freudenheim J et al. Premenopausal breast cancer risk and intake of vegetables, fruits, and related nutrients. *Journal of the National Cancer Institute,* March 1966; 88:340–348.

Friedman G. *Primer of Epidemiology.* New York: McGraw-Hill, 1974.

Gaddi A et al. Dietary treatment for familial hyperchlesterolemia—differential effects of dietary soy protein according to the apolipoprotein E phenotypes. *American Journal of Clinical Nutrition,* May 1991; 53:1191–1196.

Garcia L et al. Differential effects of aspirin and nonsteroidal anti-inflammatory drugs in the primary prevention of myocardial infarction in postmenopausal women. *Epidemiology,* July 2000; 11:382–387.

Garg R et al. Niacin treatment increased plasma homocysteine levels. *American Heart Journal,* December 1999; 138:1082–1087.

Ginsburg E et al. Effects of alcohol ingestion on estrogen in postmenopausal women. *Journal of the American Medical Association,* December 1996; 276:1747–1751.

Ginsburg J. Lack of significant hormonal effects and controlled trials of phytooestrogens. *Lancet,* January 2000; 355:163–164.

Giovannucci E et al. Intake of fat, meat, and fiber in relation to risk of colon cancer in men. *Cancer Research,* May 1994; 54:2390–2397.

Gittleman A. *Beyond Pritikin.* New York: Bantam Books, 1988.

Goodman M et al. Association of dairy products, lactose and calcium with the risk of ovarian cancer. *American Journal of Epidemiology,* July 2002; 156:148–157.

Gottlib N. Nonhormonal agents show promise against hot flashes. *Journal of the National Cancer Institute,* July 2000; 92:1118–1120.

Grady D et al. Hormone replacement therapy to prevent diseases and prolong life in post-menopausal women. *Annals of Internal Medicine*, December 1992; 117:1016–1037.

Grady D and Cummings S. Postmenopausal hormone therapy for prevention of fractures: how good is the evidence? (editorial), *Journal of the American Medical Association*, June 2001; 285:2909–2910.

Greer G. *The Change*. New York: Fawcett Columbine, 1991.

Haas R. *Permanent Remission*. New York: Pocket Books, 1997.

Haffner et al. Reduced coronary events in simvastatin-treated patients with coronary heart disease and diabetes or impaired fasting glucose levels: subgroup analysis in the Scandinavian Simvastatin Survival Study. *Archives of Internal Medicine*, December 1999; 159:2661–2667.

Hahn N. Are phytoestrogens natures' cure for what ails us? A look at the research. *Journal of the American Dietetic Association*, September 1998; 98:974–976.

Hamajima N et al. Alcohol, tobacco and breast cancer–collaborative reanalysis of individual data from 53 epidemiological studies, including 58,525 women with breast cancer and 95,067 women without the disease. *British Journal of Cancer*, November 2002; 87:1234–1245.

Harkness G. *Epidemiology in Nursing Practice*. St. Louis: Mosby-Year Book, Inc., 1995.

Hebert P et al. Cholesterol lowering with statin drugs, risk of stroke, and total mortality. An overview of randomized trials. *Journal of the American Medical Association*, July 1997; 278:313–321.

Heinonen O et al. The Helsinki Heart Study: coronary heart disease incidence during an extended follow-up. *Journal of Internal Medicine*, January 1994; 235: 41–49.

Hennessy S and Storm B. Statins and fracture risk (editorial). *Journal of the American Medical Association*. April 2001; 285:1888–1889.

Hively W. The mathematics of making up your mind. *Discover*, May 1996:90–97.

Holland E et al. Changes in collagen composition and cross-linking in bone and skin of osteoporotic postmenopausal women treated with percutaneous estradiol implants. *Obstetrics and Gynecolog,y*, February 1994; 83:180–183.

Homocysteine Studies Collaboration. Homocysteine and risk of ischemic heart disease and stroke. *Journal of the American Medical Association*, October 2002; 288:2015–2022.

House J et al. Social relationships and health. *Science*, July 1988; 241:540–545.

Hu F et al. Dietary saturated fats and their food sources in relation to the risk of coronary heart disease in women. *American Journal of Clinical Nutrition*, December 1999; 70:1001–1008.

Hu F et al. Frequent nut consumption and risk of coronary heart disease in women: prospective cohort study. *British Medical Journal*, November 1998; 317:1341–1345.

Hu F et al. Physical activity and risk of stoke in women. *Journal of the American Medical*, June 2000; 283:2961–2967.

Iribarren C et al. Association of hostility with coronary artery calcification in young adults: the CARDIA study. Coronary Artery Risk Development Young Adults. *Journal of the American Medical Association*, May 2000; 283:2546–2551.

Jardin B et al. Dietary factors associated with breast and prostate cancer development. *Journal of Nutrition* (review), November 2002; 132:3544S(2).

Jiang R et al. Nut and peanut butter consumption and risk of type 2 diabetes in women. *Journal of the American Medical Association*, November 2002; 288:2554–2560.

Kennedy A. The evidence for soybean products as cancer preventive agents. *Journal of Nutrition*, 1995; 1225:733s–743S.

Khosla P and Hayes K. Dietary trans-monounsaturated fatty acids negatively impact plasma lipids in humans: critical review of the evidence. *Journal of the American College of Nutrition*, August 1996; 15:325–339.

Klerk M et al. MTHFR 677C→T polymorphism and risk of coronary heart disease. *Journal of the American Medical Association*, October 2002; 288:2023–2031.

Lamartiniere, C et al. Genistein suppresses mammary cancer in rats. *Carcinogenesis*, 1995; 16:2833–2840.

LaRosa J et al. Effects of statins on risk of coronary disease: a meta-analysis of randomized controlled trials. *Journal of the American Medical Association*, December 2000; 282:2340–2346.

Lavoie K and Fleet R. The impact of depression on the course and outcome of coronary artery disease review for cardiologists. *Canandian Journal of Cardiology*, May 2000; 16:653–652.

Law M et al. By how much and how quickly does reduction in serum cholesterol concentration lower risk of ischaemic heart disease? *Bristish Medical Journal*, February 1994; 308:367–372.

Lee J. *What Your Doctor May Not Tell You About Menopause*. New York: Warner Books, 1996.

Libby P. Atherosclerosis: The New View. *Scientific American*, May 2002; 286:47–53.

Libby P et al. Roles of infectious agents in atheroscleroiss and restenosis: an assessment of the evidence and need for future research. *Circulation*, December 1997; 96:4095–4103.

Lin S et al. Whole-grain consumption and risk of coronary heart disease: results from the Nurses' Health Study. *American Journal of Clinical Nutrition* September 1999; 70:412–419.

Lock M et al. Cultural construction of menopause: the Japanese case. *Maturitas*, June 1988; 10:317–332.

Love S. *Dr. Susan Love's Hormone Book*. New York: Random House, 1997.

Mackenzie I et al. Anti-inflamatory drugs and alzheimer-type pathology in aging. *Neurology*, February 2000; 54:732–734.

Mamburg M. *Basic Statistics*. New York: Harcourt Brace Jovanovich, 1979.

Maricic M. Early prevention vs late treatment for osteoporosis. *Archives of Internal Medicine* December 1997; 157:2545–2546.

Marks R. *Analyzing Research Data*. London: Lifetime Learning Publications, 1982.

Martin M et al. Menopause without symptoms: the endocrinology of menopause among rural Mayan Indians. *American Journal of Obstetrics and Gynecology*, June 1993; 168:1839–1845.

Mateo K and Kirchhoff K. *Using and Conducting Nursing Research in the Clinical Setting*. Philadelphia: W.B Saunders, 1999.

Matthews D and Farewell V. *Using and Understanding Medical Statistics*. New York: Karger, 1988.

Mausner J and Bahn A. *Epidemiology*. Philadelphia: W.B. Saunders, 1974.

McCance K and Huether S. *Pathophysiology: the Biologic Basis for Disease and Adults and Children*. St. Louis: C.V. Mosby Co., 1990.

Mercuri M et al. Pravastatin reduces carotid intima-media thickness progression in an asymptomatic hypercholesterolemic mediterranan population: The Carotid

Atherosclerosis Italian Ultrasound Study. *American Journal of Medicine*, December 1996; 101:627–634.

Messina M et al. The role of soy products in reducing risk of cancer. *Journal of the National Cancer Institute*, April 1991; 83:541–546.

Miettinen et al. Cholesterol-lowering therapy in women and elderly patients with myocardial infarction or angina pectoris, findings from the Scandinavian Simvastatin Survival Study (4S). *Circulation*, December 1997; 96:4211–4218.

Morris J. *Uses of Epidemiology*. New York: Churchill Livingstone, 1975.

Morrison H et al. Serum folate and risk of fatal coronary heart disease. *Journal of the American Medical Association*, June 1996; 275:1893–1896.

Morton R and Hekel J. *A Study Guide to Epidemiology and Biostatistics*. Baltimore: University Park Press, 1984.

Newcomb D and Trentham-Dietz A. Breast feeding practices in relation to endometrial cancer risk, USA. *Cancer Causes Control*, August 2000; 11:663–667.

Nygård O et al. Plasma homocysteine levels and mortality in patients with coronary artery disease. *The New England Journal of Medicine*, July 1997; 337:230–236.

Ojeda L. *Menopause Without Medicine*. Almeda: Hunter House, 1995.

Ornish D. *Dr. Dean Ornish's Program for Reversing Heart Disease*. New York: Random House, 1990.

Ornish D. *Eat More Weigh Less*. New York: Harper Collins, 1993.

Ornish D et al. Intensive lifestyle changes for reversal of coronary heart disease. *Journal of American Medical Association*, December 1998; 280:2001–2007.

Page H, Schroeder J, and Dickson T. *The Standford Life Plan for a Healthy Heart*. San Francisco: Chronicle Books, 1996.

Pederson T et al. (for the Scandinavian Simvastatin Survival Study). Randomized trial of cholesterol lowering in 4444 patients with coronary heart disease: the Scandinavian Simvastatin Survival Study (4s). *The Lancet*, November 1994; 344: 1383–1389.

Pedersen T et al. Statin trials and goals of cholesterol-lowering therapy after AML. *American Heart Journal*, August 1999; 138:177–182.

Plotnick G et al. Effects of antioxidant vitamins on the transient impairment of endothelium-dependent brachial artery vasoactivity following a single high-fat meal. *Journal of the American Medical Association*, November 1997; 278:1682–1686.

Pritikin R. *The New Pritikin Program*. New York: Pocket Books, 1990.

Reichmann J. *I'm Too Young to Get Old*. New York: Times Books, 1997.

Reis L. et al. *SEER Cancer Statistical Review*, 1973–1999 (Tables and Graphs), National Cancer Institute. National Institute of Health (NIH) Publishing: Bethesda, Maryland.

Researchers for the Cancer and Steroid Hormone Study of the Centers for Disease Control and the National Institute of Child Health and Human Development. Combination oral contraceptive use and the risk of endometrial cancer. *Journal of the American Medical Association*, February 1987; 257:796–800.

Ridker P et al. C-reactive protein adds to the predictive value of total and HDL cholesterol in determining risk of first myocardial infarction. *Circulation*, May 1998; 97:2007–2011.

Ridker P et al. (For the CARE investigators): Inflammation, prevastatin and the risk of coronary events after myocardial infarction in patients with average cholesterol levels. *Circulation*, September 1998; 98:839–844.

Rimm E et al. Moderate alcohol intake and lower risks of coronary heart disease: meta-analysis of effects on lipids and haemostatic factors. *British Medical Journal*, December 1999; 319:1523–1528.

Rimm E et al. Review of moderate alcohol consumption and reduced risk of coronary heart disease: is the effect due to beer, wine, or spirits? *British Medical Journal*, December 1996; 312:731–736.

Rose D. The mechanistic rationale in support of dietary cancer prevention. *Preventive Medicine*, Jan.–Feb.1996; 25:34–37.

Rosen C. Restoring aging bones. *Scientific American*, March 2003; 288:70–77.

Runyon R. *Fundamentals of Statistics in the Biological, Medical and Health Sciences.* Boston: Duxbury Press, 1985.

Sarkkinen E et al. Long-term effect of three fat-modified diets in hypercholestrolemic subjects. *Atherosclerosis*, January 1994; 105:9–23.

Schaefer E et al. Lipoprotein (a) levels and risk of coronary heart disease in men. The Lipid Research Clinics Coronary Primary Prevention Trial. *Journal of the American Medical Association*, April 1994; 271:999–1003.

Schah P et al. Circulating markers of inflammation for vascular risk prediction are they ready for prime time. *Circulation*, April 2000; 101:1758–1759.

Schlesselman J. *Case-Control Studies.* New York: Oxford Press, 1982.

Schneeman B. Dietary Influences on Health. *Preventive Medicine*, Jan–Feb. 1996; 25:38–40.

Schnyder G et al. Effects of homocysteine-lowering therapy with folic acid, vitamin B12, and vitamin B6 on clinical outcome after percutaneous coronary intervention (The Swiss Heart Study). *Journal of the American Medical Association*, August 2002; 288:973–979.

Senti M, Aubo C, and Tomas M. Differential effects of smoking on myocardial infarction risk according to the Gln/Arg 192 variants of the human paraoxonase gene. *Metabolism*, May 2000; 49:557–559.

Singletary K and Gapstur S. Alcohol and breast cancer: review of epidemiologic and experimental evidence and potential mechanism. Journal of the American Medical Association, November 2001; 286:2143.

Sirtori C et al. Aortic and coronary atheromatosis in a woman with severe hypercholesterolaemia without LDL receptor alterations. *European Heart Journal*, July 1991; 12:818–824.

Sirtori C et al. Double-blind study of the additon of high-protein soya milk v.cows' milk to the diet of patients with severe hypercholesterolaemia and resistance to or intolerance of statins. *British Journal of Nutrition*, August 1999; 82:91–96.

Sirtori C et al. Olive oil., Corn oil, and n-3 fatty acids differently affect lipids, lipoproteins, platlets, and superoxide formation in type II hypercholesterolemia. *American Journal of Clinical Nutrition*, July 1992; 56:113–122.

Stampfer M et al. Primary prevention of coronary heart disease in women through diet and lifestyle. *The New England Journal of Medicine*, July 2000; 343:16–22.

Stanford J and Thomas D. Exogenous progestins and breast cancer. *Epidemiologic Reviews*, April 1993; 15:98–107.

Stark R. Review of the major intervention trials of lowering coronary artery disease risk through cholesterol reduction. *American Journal of Cardiology*, September 1996; 78:13–19.

Stein F. *Anatomy of Clinical Research.* Thorofare: SLACK Inc., 1989.

Steinberg K et al. A meta-analysis of the effect of estrogen replacement therapy on the risk of breast cancer. *Journal of the American Medical Association*, April 1991; 265:1985–1990.

Tang J et al. Systematic review of dietary intervention trials to lower blood total cholesterol in free-living subjects. *British Medical Journal*, April 1998; 316:1213–1220.

Trosi R et al. Insulin and endometrial cancer. *American Journal of Epidemiology*, September 1997; 146:476–482.

Valanis B. *Epidemiology in Nursing and Health Care*. Norwalk: Appleton & Lange, 1992.

van Staa T et al. Use of statins and risk of fractures. *Journal of the American Medical Association*, April 2001; 285:1850–1855.

Verhoef P et al. Homocysteine metabolism and risk of myocardial infarction: relation with vitamins B6, B12, and folate. *American Journal of Epidemiology*, May 1996; 143:845–859.

Wilcox G et al. Oestrogen effects of plant foods on postmenopausal women. *British Medical Journal*, October 1991; 301:905–906.

Willett W and Stamper M. Rebuilding the food pyramid. *Scientific American*, January 2003; 288:65–71.

Willett W et al. Dietary fat and the risk of breast cancer. *The New England Journal of Medicine*, 1987; 316:22–28.

Willett W et al. Intake of trans fatty acids and risk of coronary heart disease among women. *Lancet*, March 1993; 341:581–585.

Willett W et al. Postmenopausal estrogens—opposed, unopposed, or none of the above. *Journal of the American Medical Association*, January 2000; 283:534–535.

Willett W et al. Trans fatty acids: are the effects only marginal? *American Journal of Public Health*, May 1994; 84:722–724.

Zhang J and Yu K. What's the relative risk? a method of correcting the odds ratio in cohort studies of common outcome. *Journal of the American Medical Association*, November 1998; 280:1690–1691.

<http://www.american.heart.org
<http://www.cancer.gov
<http://www.meds.com
<http://www.nci.nih.gov
<http://www.seer.cancer.gov

Index